newest ed.
11/2013 gm

Date Due

JUN 3 0 2004			
	DISCARDED		

Physiotherapy for Amputees

For Churchill Livingstone

Publisher: Mary Law
Project Editor: Dinah Thom
Copy Editor: Prunella Theaker
Production Controller: Mark Sanderson
Sales Promotion Executive: Hilary Brown

Physiotherapy for Amputees
The Roehampton Approach

Barbara Engstrom MCSP CertMHS

Superintendent Physiotherapist
University College and Middlesex Hospitals
London

Catherine Van de Ven MCSP

District Physiotherapist
Richmond, Twickenham & Roehampton Health Authority
Queen Mary's University Hospital
Roehampton Lane
London

Illustrations by Jane Upton

SECOND EDITION

CHURCHILL LIVINGSTONE
EDINBURGH LONDON MADRID MELBOURNE NEW YORK AND TOKYO 1993

CHURCHILL LIVINGSTONE
Medical Division of Longman Group UK Limited

Distributed in the United States of America by Churchill
Livingstone Inc., 650 Avenue of the Americas, New York,
N.Y. 10011, and by associated companies, branches and
representatives throughout the world.

First edition 1985
Second edition 1993

ISBN 0-443-04396-5

British Library Cataloguing in Publication Data
A catalogue record for this book is available from the British
Library.

Library of Congress Cataloging in Publication Data
Engstrom, Barbara.
    Physiotherapy for amputees: the Roehampton approach/Barbara
Engstrom, Catherine Van de Ven; illustrations by J. Upton. — 2nd ed.
        p.   cm.
    Includes bibliographical references and index.
    ISBN 0-443-04396-5
    1. Amputees—Rehabilitation.   2. Physical therapy. I. Van de
Ven, Catherine. II. Title.
    [DNLM: 1. Amputees—rehabilitation.   2. Physical Therapy.   WE 172
E58p]
RD553.E54   1993
617.5'8062—dc20
DNLM/DLC
for Library of Congress   92-49144

The
publisher's
policy is to use
paper manufactured
from sustainable forests

Produced by Longman Singapore Publishers (Pte) Ltd.
Printed in Singapore

Contents

Preface to the second edition

Many changes have prompted us to revise the first edition.

Firstly, changes in the legislation and organisation of the National Health Service in the UK have resulted in the need for a more flexible and adaptable approach towards amputee management. These changes are ongoing and span across the acute episode in the hospital setting and care in the community setting.

Secondly, prosthetic and wheelchair supply and management have altered significantly following the McColl Report of 1986, allowing a more flexible service for the amputee's individual needs. Smaller companies are supplying a greater variety of prostheses: new designs and components are constantly being made available and will increase as the European Common Market and world markets expand. There is now a separation between prosthetic services companies and the manufacturers of components and hardware. There is no longer a national overview of the service, as it is now provided for either on a regional or local basis.

Thirdly, training, education, quality and standards issues are now also addressed at local level.

This second edition addresses some of these aspects and aims to help the clinical physiotherapist to cope with this constantly changing scene by paying attention to basic principles. It is still intended as a handbook for qualified and student physiotherapists and as such is still practically orientated. However, now more than ever physiotherapists must read more widely, paying attention to current literature including technical data concerning new prostheses, surgical techniques and rehabilitation research.

Many of our previous contributors have further assisted us; however, some no longer work in the amputee and prosthetic services but much of their original contribution remains in the text. The following people have supported us and contributed to this second edition:

For prosthetic rehabilitation services: Mrs Penny Buttenshaw MCSP, Mrs Jane Dolman MCSP, Mrs Sara Smith MCSP, Mrs Lise Robinson MCSP, Dr. S Sooriakamaran MB BS LRCP MRCS FRCS (Eng Edin & Glasg) Consultant in Rehabilitation, all from Richmond, Twickenham & Roehampton Health Authority; Ms Pam Barsby MCSP and Dr Linda Marks MRCP, Consultant in Rehabilitation, Royal National Orthopaedic Hospital Trust; Mr Peter Lewis FBIST, Mr Tony Morris FBIST, from C. A. Blatchford & Sons Ltd; Mr Barry Fazackerely FBIST, Hugh Steepers Ltd. Mr Paul Jamieson BSc, for photographic assistance from C. A. Blatchford & Sons Ltd.

Miss Fiona Carnegie DipCOT, who has revised Chapter 17 on upper limb amputation, and Miss Bridget Davis ONC MCSP, Kings Health Care, for suggestions on gait rehabilitation; Mrs Vicky Frampton MCSP, Canterbury and Thanet Health Authority, for further information on the aspects of pain and its control.

Miss Shamsie Sharmin SRCh MChS DipPodM, for further information on chiropody, and Mrs Sandra Rigling RGN, for foot care advice and diabetes, both from Richmond, Twickenham & Roehampton Health Authority.

Ms Helen Alper, Librarian, Queen Mary's University Hospital, for a literature search, the

Medical Photography Department, Queen Mary's University Hospital, and Steve Parapian, Medical Photography Department, University College and Middlesex School of Medicine, Mrs Mo Lay, Physiotherapy Department Co-ordinator, Queen Mary's University Hospital, and Miss Sonia Skinner, University College Hospital, for secretarial support.

Dr M. F. R. Waters OBE FRCP FRCPath, Consultant Leprologist, Hospital for Tropical Diseases; Mr Arthur Day OBE for assisting and coordinating much of the revised text; Liz Crowder, Product specialist of Nomeq, for her technical help.

Lastly, but equally important, the voluntary organisations who have given so much assistance:
NALD
BLESMA
STEPS
BSAD
REACH.

London, 1993   B.E.
                                                C.V.de V.

Preface to the first edition

This is intended as a handbook for both qualified and student physiotherapists in the UK and abroad. Its purpose is to impart theoretical and practical knowledge, which can be used as a basic reference for those treating and caring for amputees during all stages of rehabilitation.

We have deliberately given a step-by-step approach because we feel this may simplify some of the complications encountered daily by patients and clinical staff. This may be criticised by those concerned with physiotherapy education, but we hope this book will provide advice for immediate and effective treatments in the clinical situation. This is particularly important during the prosthetic stages of rehabilitation, as it is essential to know how and where to obtain immediate assistance.

The majority of chapters are heavily illustrated to clarify procedures and activities. After each chapter there is a list of references, and there is also a general bibliography in the Appendix to permit the reader to deepen and widen existing knowledge. We have endeavoured to make these references as international and varied as possible. We have also included a list of useful addresses and a glossary of terms in the Appendix.

The contents of this book are our ideas and suggestions based on our experiences which we have found successful over the years at Queen Mary's Hospital and the DHSS Limb Fitting Centre at Roehampton but, of course, each patient and situation must be approached individually.

We are most grateful to have been helped by many different professions in order to present an overall view of the Roehampton approach. Unfortunately, we cannot mention everybody by name, but we would like to thank the following,

without whom this book would not have been possible:

Dr R. Redhead MB BS MRCS PhD, Senior Medical Officer, DHSS LFC, Roehampton, and Mrs F. Turner MCSP DipTP DipBioMech MPhil, who have read each chapter and given professional advice and assistance at all stages. Miss P. Langford MCSP and Mr J. Sim BA MCSP, who have commented on its clarity and understanding. Mr T. R. Frost FBIST, Chief Prosthetist, J. E. Hanger and Co. Ltd and Mrs D. Dixey MCSP, who have given specific advice on much of the contents.

Our main contributors: Miss A. Mendez OBE FCOT, former District Occupational Therapist, Richmond, Twickenham & Roehampton Health Authority, who has compiled and written Chapter 17; Miss A. Zigmond SRN CQSW, who has supplied written advice on social work and the psychological needs of the amputee; Mrs V. Long MChS SRCh, who has advised us on chiropody services.

Mrs J. Upton DipAD ATD, our illustrator, who has worked with us since the book's inception; much of the meaning of this book would be lost without her clear and accurate illustrations.

Mr N. Babbage, consultant photographer, Bioengineering Centre, University College, London, for his excellent photographic work. Mrs W. Bevan, Librarian, Bioengineering Centre, who has helped us search the literature.

Other professional help and advice has been supplied by the following, from Queen Mary's Hospital, Roehampton: Dr I. H. M. Curwen MB ChB DPhysMed, former Consultant in Rheumatology and Rehabilitation, Mr B. G.

Andrews FRCS, Consultant Orthopaedic Surgeon, Mr K. P. Robinson MS FRCSE FRCS, Consultant Surgeon, Dr P. Tidman MB BS FFARCS, Consultant Anaesthetist, Mr R. Ballard BSc FRCSEd MRCOG, Consultant Gynaecologist & Obstetrician, Mrs J. Hodder MCSP, Superintendent Physiotherapist, and Miss J. Jackson DipN, formerly ward sister, Limb Surgery Unit.

Dr N. Mustapha FRCS, Senior Medical Officer, Limb Fitting Service and Honorary Consultant to Queen Mary's Hospital, Dr D. J. Thornberry FRCS, and Mrs S. Riglin SRN, at DHSS LFC, Roehampton. Dr M. Dewer BSc PhD, Bioengineering Centre, University College, London, Dr J. Connolly MB MPhil FRCP FRCPsych, Consultant Psychiatrist, Maudsley Hospital, London, and Miss J. Guymer MCSP DipTP, Westminster Hospital, London. Mr M. Hammond supplied much of the information on sports for the amputee.

Mrs P. Ridgley, Manager, DHSS LFC, Roehampton, and many of her staff who have provided clerical assistance, in particular Mrs B. Spencer. Additional clerical help has been provided by Mrs C. O'Leary and Mrs M. Pretty.

Queen Mary's Roehampton Hospital Trust, and Mr J. Williams MBE, Clerk to the Trustees, for their financial help towards secretarial costs. Mrs G. Smith for her secretarial help in typing the final manuscript.

Miss S. M. Adams MCSP, District Physiotherapist, Richmond, Twickenham & Roehampton Health District, for her unfailing support and encouragement to us both during the production of this book and over the years. Also, the staff of the physiotherapy department, Queen Mary's Hospital, Roehampton, who have tried out the instructions for the functional activities and commented on them. The staff of Churchill Livingstone, for their help and advice.

We acknowledge permission to use photographs, illustrations and technical data of products of J. E. Hanger & Co. Ltd, C. A. Blatchford & Co., Vessa Ltd, Hugh Steeper (Roehampton) Ltd, and John Drew (London) Ltd. In particular, we would like to thank Mr B. O'Brien FBIST, and Mr R. Harrison LBIST, for prosthetic advice.

Lastly, but most importantly, we should like to thank all our patients, who, over the years, have taught us so much.

London, 1985

B.E.
C.V.deV.

1. Introduction

THE HISTORY OF AMPUTATIONS AND PROSTHESES

Archaeological evidence has shown that amputations were carried out as early as the Neolithic period with knives and bone saws, and skeletal remains with amputated bone stumps have been found.

In the latter half of the fifth century B.C., Hippocrates wrote a treatise 'On Joints' in which amputation for vascular gangrene and cautery was described. In the first century A.D., Celsus recommended that amputation should be between the healthy and the gangrenous tissues. There was an extremely high mortality rate brought about through shock and haemorrhage. The only forms of anaesthesia were wine and other alcoholic beverages and two assistants were needed to hold the patient down.

Ambroise Paré (1510–1590), the father of French surgery, improved ligation of large vessels during surgery and was vitally interested in the rehabilitation of the amputee, designing and manufacturing several prostheses for both upper and lower extremities. Ancient prostheses were very sophisticated by modern standards but were bulky and heavy. Many of the principles of modern prosthetics were developed and applied during this time.

The discovery of the circulation of the blood by Harvey in 1616 led to the invention of more efficient tourniquets, but speed of surgery was still essential. By the eighteenth century, better soft tissue coverage of bone ends with muscle flaps was achieved, but wound infection was frequent and often devastating. The modern concept of nursing was developed by Florence Nightingale during the Crimean War (1854–1856) in response to insanitary conditions in military hospitals. She replaced hospital chaos, filth and sorrow with scientific cleanliness, orderliness and increased well-being.

The development of anaesthesia in 1846 and Lister's aseptic technique in 1867 are the hallmarks of modern surgery. By the end of the nineteenth century the concept of allowing those muscles remaining to power the prosthesis was introduced. Prostheses at this time were fashioned out of wood. The Marquis of Anglesey, who lost his leg at the Battle of Waterloo, had a wooden prosthesis made for him by James Potts, and even today this type of prosthesis is still made and is called the Anglesey Leg.

THE HISTORY OF QUEEN MARY'S UNIVERSITY HOSPITAL, ROEHAMPTON

During the First World War, it soon became apparent that many men would survive their injuries and remain maimed by the loss of one or more limbs. In fact by 1918 over 41 000 British ex-servicemen had become amputees.

Lady Falmouth and Mrs G. Holford campaigned for the supply of artificial limbs to these men and a facility for their rehabilitation. Roehampton House, a Queen Anne mansion belonging to Kenneth Wilson, was leased by him, rent free, as a hospital. Her Majesty, Queen Mary, lent her name to the project and became one of the patrons of Queen Mary's Convalescent Auxiliary Hospital for Limbless Soldiers and Sailors which opened in June 1915. Over half the total number of amputees from the First World War were treated at Roehampton. J. F. Rowley was given the contract

1

to set up a factory on the same site as the hospital for the manufacture of artificial limbs. This was later taken over by J. E. Hanger & Co. (The history of the limb fitting service is covered in Ch. 7.)

In 1925 the hospital became known as Queen Mary's Hospital, Roehampton, and started admitting civilian amputees. It was then administered by the Ministry of Pensions until 1960 when it was transferred to the Westminster Hospital Board of Governors. During the Second World War there were fewer amputees and more war disabled patients were treated. In 1948, as a result of the National Health Service Act, an increased number of non ex-service patients were treated. It is at present the district general hospital of the Richmond, Twickenham & Roehampton Health Authority and its specialist disability services remain on site.

STATISTICS OF THE PRESENT-DAY AMPUTEE POPULATION

In England and Wales there is an amputee population of 66 600 (53 405 lower limb and 13 196 upper limb). However, this is not the total number as it only reflects those referred to a limb fitting centre. There are approximately 5000 new amputees referred to regional disablement services centres in England and Wales each year (Table 1.1). These 1985 statistics were the last national figures: more recent statistics are collected on a regional basis. Separate statistics are kept in Scotland at the Scottish Home and Health Department. The ratio of male to female is about 2:1, and the ratio of lower to upper limbs is about 24:1.

Over 80% of patients having a leg amputated suffer from vascular disease (see Table 1.2), and the majority are older than 60 years of age. This type of patient presents with the many and varied medical problems of the elderly and so requires detailed care and forethought in rehabilitative management.

Table 1.1 First time attendance 1985 in limb fitting centres in England and Wales

Single leg	4797
Double leg	457
Single arm	332
Double arm	3
	5589

Table 1.2 Indications for amputation of a leg 1985

Vascular	60.3 %
Diabetic	21 %
Trauma	9 %
Malignancy	4.5 %
Infective	1.5 %
Congenital defect	3.6 %

About 10% of new leg amputees are as a result of trauma, half of these being through road traffic accidents. Most of these patients are young and may have multiple injuries. This type of patient not only requires effective, speedy and progressive rehabilitative treatment, but also much psychological help and skilled counselling.

Malignancy accounts for about 5% of new leg amputees each year; the majority are children and teenagers whose life expectancy is low. Their management by everyone involved must be speedy; at the same time considerable psychological support must be given to the parents.

Arm amputations are mainly performed as a result of accidents. Table 1.3 gives full details of these. A few amputees are patients with congenital abnormalities of either upper or lower limbs, who elect to have an amputation for both cosmetic and functional reasons.

AMPUTATION SURGERY

In the UK, amputation surgery is normally carried out in district general hospitals. The patient is usually under the care of the vascular, general surgery or orthopaedic consultant.

Levels of amputation

There are certain levels of amputation which provide a stump suitable for prosthetic fitting, function and cosmesis. It is essential that one of these levels is selected rather than the boundary

Table 1.3 Indications for amputation of an arm 1985

Accident (RTA, home, recreation, etc)	37.6 %
Industrial accident	25 %
Malignancy	22.3 %
Embolism	6.6 %
Other vascular disease	4.3 %
Deformity	1.6 %
Metabolic disorders/infection	2.6 %

of the dead or diseased tissue with the viable (Figs 1.1 and 1.2).

PHILOSOPHY OF THE AMPUTATION SERVICE

Every patient is an individual and must always be considered within the context of their particular abilities, medical and environmental status, never as a 'level'.

At Roehampton, work with amputees has progressed for many years in varying circumstances. The approach has been developed through constant observation and practical handling of many different types of patient. Research has provided even greater insight into these amputees' problems and thus given a wider understanding of the total overall management.

The Roehampton model has been accepted and developed in other centres and involves caring for the patient at all stages, i.e. from the pre-operative stage to discharge, when the patient is fully mobile with a prosthesis or a wheelchair or both, and with community links and subsequent long-term follow-up. In order to achieve this, a large team of professionals work with each other towards a common end. In addition to the patient and their relatives, the team consists of:

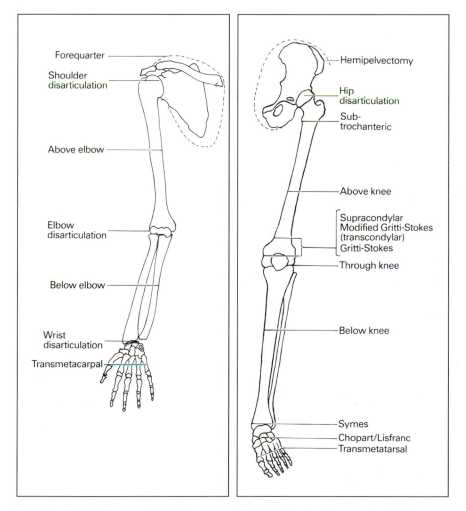

Fig. 1.1 Levels of amputation in the upper limb.

Fig. 1.2 Levels of amputation in the lower limb.

— Surgeon
— Rehabilitation consultant
— Nurse
— Physiotherapist
— Occupational therapist
— Social worker
— Prosthetist
— Rehabilitation engineer.

This team meets regularly for ward rounds, or for group case discussion, problem solving and forward planning. Every member of the team has an equal opportunity to present his or her thoughts which contribute to the group decision on patient management.

Additional consultation:

— Rheumatology consultant
— General physician
— Geriatrician
— Any other hospital consultant as required
— General practitioner (GP)
— Dietician
— Chiropodist
— Local Authority Social Service Department
— Speech therapist
— Disablement resettlement officer (DRO)
— Clinical psychologist
— Nurse counsellor
— Hospital chaplaincy service
— Bioengineer
— Orthotist.

The physiotherapist is in a unique position, being involved practically with the patient's management at all stages, both pre- and post-operatively, during mobility training with a prosthesis or wheelchair, and in the home. The physiotherapist continues to treat the amputee's problems as they arise, and this must be thorough and, at times, persistent, so that the greatest potential can be achieved. Anything less than daily treatment of amputees is unacceptable.

The team as a whole accepts that not all amputees are able to cope with prosthetic rehabilitation, and wheelchair independence or other forms of mobility for this group is a positive functional achievement. The quality of a patient's remaining life must be considered, and lengthy prosthetic rehabilitation is contra-indicated in some instances.

In some centres there is an ideal situation with disability services on the same site as the acute hospital, enabling easier communication. However, facilities may not all be in such close proximity, but communication between the many professionals involved is crucial and may require considerable personal effort.

Additional facilities available at Roehampton

1. *Combined clinic.* Patients can be sent to this clinic from all over Great Britain by consultants, GPs and doctors from disability centres, for consultation prior to amputation, or revision to another level of amputation. The patient is seen by a consultant orthopaedic surgeon and the rehabilitation consultant.

2. *Limb surgery unit.* This is a 12 bedded ward opened in 1974; it is used for adult amputation surgery and subsequent rehabilitation.

3. *The Leon Gillis Centre.* This was originally designed for thalidomide children and was opened in 1963; it has now diversified into the management of children suffering from all types of abnormalities. It is a multidisciplinary unit, providing assessment and treatment for severely handicapped children. Children from birth to 18 years of age are accepted; support and help are also available for the parents.

4. *The district wheelchair service.* The local wheelchair service is based on the hospital site offering regular assessment clinics for basic wheelchair needs.

5. *Regional wheelchair service.* This is a specialised service using a multidisciplinary approach with specific expertise in seating and more complex equipment.

REFERENCES

Dallas Brodie I A O 1970 Lower limb amputation. British Medical Journal 4: 596–604

Department of Health and Social Security Statistics and Research Division 1985 Amputation statistics for England, Wales and N. Ireland

English A W G, Gregory Dean A A 1980 The artificial limb service. Health Trends 12: 77

Glattly H W 1964 Statistical study of 12 000 new amputees. Southern Medical Journal 57: 1373–1378

Glattly H W 1968 Preliminary report on amputee census. Artificial Limbs 7: 5–10

Ham R, Thornberry D J, Regan J C et al 1985 Rehabilitation of the vascular amputee — one method evaluated. Physiotherapy Practice 1: 6–13

Ham R, Van de Ven C 1986 The management of the lower limb amputee in England and Wales today. Physiotherapy Practice 2: 94–100

Kay H W, Newman J D 1974 Amputee survey 1973–74; preliminary findings and comparisons. Orthotics and Prosthetics 28(2): 27–32

Knight P, Urquhart J 1989 Outcomes of artificial lower limb fitting in Scotland. Information and Statistics Division, Common Services Agency for the Scottish Health Service, Edinburgh

McColl I 1986 Review of artificial limb and appliance centre services. DHSS, London, vols 1 & 2

Murdoch G 1977 Amputation surgery in the lower extremity. Prosthetics and Orthotics International 1: 72–83

Murdoch G 1984 Amputation revisited. Prosthetics and Orthotics International 8: 8–15

Narang I C, Jape V S 1982 Retrospective study of 14 400 civilian disabled (new) treated over 25 years at an Artificial Limb Centre. Prosthetics and Orthotics International 6: 10–16

Orr J R, James W V, Bahrani A S 1982 The history and development of artificial limbs. Engineering in Medicine 11(4): 155–161

Robins R 1984 An old Cornish hand. Journal of Hand Surgery 98: 199–200

Robinson K P 1980 Limb ablation and limb replacement. Annals of the Royal College of Surgeons of England 62: 87–105

2. Pre-operative assessment

The physiotherapist's pre-operative assessment is concerned with the physical state of the patient, the social situation and home environment.

Following a diagnosis by the doctor, the physiotherapist will relate the assessment of the patient to the implications of that diagnosis:

a. to evaluate the patient's physical and psychological status
b. to evaluate the affected limb
c. to initiate a programme of action required to facilitate future rehabilitation.

CONDITIONS PREDISPOSING TO AMPUTATION

Each of the following conditions has important aspects which need to be considered by the physiotherapist:

1. Vascular disease — atherosclerosis
2. Vascular disease — diabetes mellitus
3. Trauma
4. Tumour
5. Congenital deformity.

Vascular disease — atherosclerosis

Atherosclerosis is a disease of the arterial system. Plaques of atheroma can be deposited in any artery of the body, for example:

— Cerebral atheroma can cause cerebrovascular accidents
— Myocardial atheroma can cause myocardial infarction
— Mesenteric atheroma can cause infarction of the gut
— Peripheral vascular disease can cause limb ischaemia.

Therefore, it must be remembered that, although the presenting problem may be one of a gangrenous foot, the patient can also be suffering from vascular disease elsewhere in the body. Patients can complain of intermittent claudication and there may be open sore areas around the toes or heel. The appearance of the skin is hairless, shiny, and the colour can be white, red or blue. Frequently, vascular reconstructive surgery can relieve these symptoms, but if the disease has progressed too far or surgery has failed, the symptoms which then bring the patient to amputation are:

a. *Gangrene*. Particularly if septicaemia is present.

b. *Rest pain*. This is intolerable ischaemic pain at rest and particularly at night. The patient does not sleep and may obtain some relief by hanging the affected limb out over the edge of the bed. This dependent position encourages blood flow to the extremity.

These two positive indications for amputation also apply to venous ulcers and Buerger's disease (this may also affect the upper limb). It is possible that the patient may already have had one leg amputated and requires further surgery to the stump or the remaining leg as the atherosclerosis progresses.

Investigations for vascular disease

a. *Clinical examination of the limb*. The general appearance and temperature of the limb is noted, together with the condition of the skin, its colour and texture. The femoral, popliteal, posterior tibial and dorsalis pedis pulses are palpated.

7

b. *Chest X-ray.*

c. *Blood tests.* Biochemical and haematological studies are carried out to detect factors which are known to increase the viscosity and hence reduce the flow of blood. The tests included are measurement of: fasting serum cholesterol, platelet abnormalities and clotting changes.

d. *Electrocardiogram.*

e. *Doppler studies.* This is a non-invasive technique which involves the application of an ultrasonic wave over an artery. This wave is beamed over a moving stream of blood, producing a frequency shift which is a function of the rate of blood flow. A pressure index can be ascertained by obtaining the ratio between systolic arterial pressure at the ankle and that in the brachial artery. Ankle pressure divided by brachial pressure is called the brachial index. A value of 1 or more excludes significant vascular disease in the lower limb. Claudication indices are 0.4–0.8, and critical ischaemia indices are as low as 0.2–0.4. Advanced forms of this investigation are laser Doppler and duplex scanning. The latter provides an image of the vessels as well as a measure of the flow in them.

f. *Arteriography.* This is an invasive technique in which radio-opaque dye is injected into the arterial system. X-rays are then taken which indicate the patency of both the main and collateral vessels. This indicates whether reconstructive surgery is possible.

g. *Venogram.* This is an X-ray of the venous system, performed in a similar manner to arteriography.

h. *Thermography.* This is a measurement of skin temperature in the whole limb, reflecting, among other factors, the level of cutaneous tissue viability, blood flow and hence the degree of ischaemia. A particular area cannot be considered in isolation but only in comparison with other areas.

i. *Transcutaneous PO_2 readings.* This is a measurement of skin oxygen pressure which reflects the level of cutaneous blood flow hence the degree of ischaemia.

Othser tests may be carried out in specialist centres with vascular laboratories, e.g. treadmill exercises, strain gauge plethysmography, Doppler, echo and duplex imaging, digital subtraction angiography, radionucleartide distraction studies, nuclear magnetic resonance, isotope clearance structure of the skin and muscle.

Advanced technology is enabling more detailed clinical investigation and will become increasingly available in district general hospitals in time.

Vascular disease — diabetes mellitus

Diabetes mellitus is a systemic disorder in which blood glucose may be intermittently raised above the normal range. The complications of diabetes may cause small blood vessel damage which can affect different parts of the body in the following ways:

— Retinopathy can lead to impairment of vision and occasionally blindness.
— Glomerulosclerosis can lead to renal failure and death.
— Neuropathy of the peripheral nerves can lead to impaired sensation in the hands and feet, the distal portion of all digits being more severely affected.
— Small artery disease can lead to peripheral or coronary ischaemia.

Healing is often poor in these patients and even minor trauma can be a major problem.

Lesions of the feet can result from impaired circulation and poor sensation. The high glucose levels in the wound encourage bacterial growth, resulting in infection which may also extend to the bone. This can lead to gangrene, and while local amputation of parts of the foot can be attempted, these may not heal and a more proximal level must then be selected.

Because of a chemical reaction, diabetics are also more prone to vascular disease in large vessels, which could lead to cerebral and coronary ischaemia and peripheral vascular disease. Many of these patients therefore have both large and small artery disease. Reconstructive vascular surgery is not always successful in the diabetic patient because of poor healing.

Investigations in diabetes

a. *Blood tests*: to estimate the blood sugar level. The normal range after 8 hours starvation is 3.3 – 5.5 mmol/l.

b. *Urine tests*: to estimate the sugar and ketone levels.

c. *Diet*: A well-balanced, high-fibre/low-fat diet is advised for diabetic patients today, rather than the rigid counting of carbohydrate units at each meal. However, each patient should seek advice from their diabetic nurse specialist or dietician, according to their individual needs.

Trauma

Amputation of a limb can either take place immediately at the site of an accident or the extensive trauma can cause sufficient damage or death of tissue to require subsequent ablation.

The aim in trauma management is to restore the lower limb to the best possible length with a good soft tissue covering. To achieve this, the expertise, cooperation and rational decision making of orthopaedic, plastic and vascular surgeons is necessary. This team must bear in mind priorities of surgical management from initial injury to successful prosthetic outcome.

In an emergency setting, life may be saved by sacrificing the limb, but once the patient has stabilised the decision concerning limb salvage and optimum level of amputation can be made. The psychological make-up of the patient and their goals and employment must be considered. The basic surgical techniques to achieve wound healing are appropriate handling of soft tissue, wound debridement, secondary wound closure and control of sepsis, and these will inevitably delay physical rehabilitation.

The amputation can therefore take place immediately, or months or even years following the trauma, and this final decision should only be taken after extensive assessment and discussion between the patient, the surgeon and the rehabilitation team (see Combined clinic, Ch. 1 p. 4).

Examples of trauma

— Compound fractures, particularly those involving skin and soft tissue loss, often in association with multiple injuries

— Blood vessel rupture
— Severe burns
— Stab, gunshot or blast wounds
— A compression injury
— Cold trauma, i.e. frostbite.

The above may occur in combination.

Investigations in trauma

a. *X-rays*. Skeletal, arteriography, venography.

b. *Estimation of skin loss*. Wallace's Rule of Nines is used for burns patients. A visual assessment of the depth and area of soft tissue loss is noted in the non-burnt patient.

c. *Clinical examination of the limb*.

d. *Assessment:*
  (i) physical
  (ii) psychological.

It is necessary to find this out by speaking to relatives and friends of the injured person.

Tumour

Patients with this condition usually present with pain or a history of trivial trauma, as a result of which an X-ray is taken and the tumour is discovered almost by chance. Sometimes there is a swelling present, but otherwise there is no other physical sign.

Primary malignant tumours of bone are rare. The most common types are osteosarcoma, chondrosarcoma, Ewing's tumour, fibrosarcoma and giant cell tumour. The majority of patients with these tumours are under 30 years of age.

In Great Britain there are two supraregional bone tumour services, in Birmingham and in London. These centres have the best facilities for investigation and treatment.

Following diagnosis of the tumour the treatment may involve chemotherapy or radiotherapy, massive excision and endoprosthetic replacement, or amputation. However, it should always be remembered that even if massive replacement is the treatment of choice, the patient may eventually come to amputation, either for recurrence of the tumour or infection in the replacement.

The physiotherapist needs to communicate with the medical oncologist, surgeon and radiotherapist monitoring each case, in order to set appropriate and realistic goals of treatment. Whatever the choice of treatment, the psychological preparation of both the patient and their parents or carers is of the utmost importance, and the clinical psychologist, psychiatrist and social worker are all involved to ensure that emotional and psychological problems are identified quickly and dealt with effectively.

The physical rehabilitation programme must be flexible to accommodate the problems of concurrent treatments. As the patients are young they can cope with extensive activity for the periods between chemotherapy. However, there are other times when no form of physiotherapy is possible.

In adult life, metastatic tumours in the skeleton are much more common than primary malignant tumours. The primary lesions are usually found in the breast, prostate gland, kidney or lung. These patients more commonly present with pain or a pathological fracture. The treatment given is usually conservative, with internal fixation of the fracture.

Investigations for tumours

a. *X-ray.* Skeletal, including bone scan, angiography and computerised axial tomography (CAT scan).
b. *MRI scan* to find extent of soft tissue involvement.
c. *Biopsy.* This is the most reliable means of diagnosis and is performed after the X-rays have determined the site of the lesion.

Congenital deformity

A child can be born with partial or complete absence of one limb, up to total absence of all four limbs, or any combination between these two extremes. There may be absence of bone, or another deformity present.

The classification of congenital limb deficiencies is complicated, and a working party set up by the International Society for Prosthetics and Orthotics (ISPO) has now produced a system of classification constructed on an anatomical basis. Deficiencies are identified as being either transverse or longitudinal.

a. *Transverse.* The limb has developed normally to a particular level beyond which no skeletal elements exist, although there may be digital buds. Some children may have several of their limbs affected, but most commonly the child presents with a single deformity at below-elbow level.

b. *Longitudinal.* There is a reduction or absence of a bone within the long axis of the limb. This will affect the development of structures distal to that bone. For example, a child with a short femur and absent tibia is likely to have absence of the lateral side of the foot as in Figure 2.1: for this child an extension prosthesis enables her to walk.

These children's problems are very complex. The child's local disablement services centre should be informed as soon after the birth as possible. Parents and children feel less isolated, gain confidence and benefit from meeting others with similar problems as readjustments for the whole family are initially quite enormous. From the centre they can be put in touch with self-help groups such as REACH and STEPS (see Appendix). Both of these organisations provide support and encouragement for parents in the first few years of their child's life.

The child's development must be monitored, and intervention, either prosthetically or surgically, should be made at the right time. It is essential that this is carried out in a specialised centre, where all the disciplines involved have a highly developed knowledge of rehabilitation in these complex cases. This can mean fitting a child's first upper limb prosthesis as early as 3 months (e.g. in the case of a single below-elbow transverse deformity). A lower limb prosthesis can be fitted between 6 and 8 months to coincide with the child's first attempts to pull itself up into standing. For children with severe lower limb abnormalities it may be necessary either to supply an extension prosthesis during the early stages of their development (see Fig. 2.1) or to amputate severely deformed limbs. This surgical decision should not be taken lightly and should only be

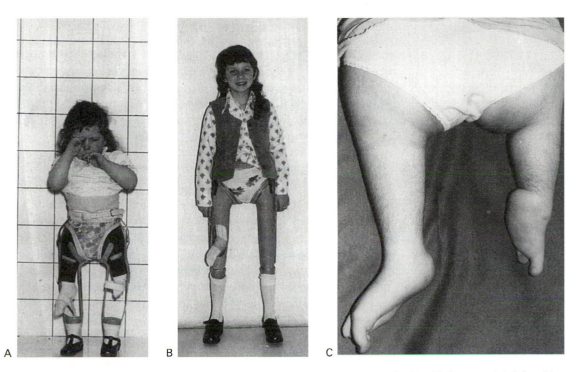

Fig. 2.1 Extension prostheses: (A) child at 3 years; (B) same child at 9 years; (C) this child's congenital deformities at 13 years.

carried out after full consultation with the rehabilitation team, including the prosthetist, the family and the child. It must be remembered that the same reaction to ablative surgery will be felt by these children as by normally developed people who undergo an amputation.

How the child will cope with disability and a prosthesis will largely depend on the parental attitude and the child's peer group. Children from a stable home who remain in the same locality generally do well as they are encouraged from an early age to socialise at play groups, nursery schools, etc. There are potential crisis points when starting school, when moving to the upper school (which is often at around the time of puberty) and when leaving school for employment or higher education. These difficult periods can be anticipated and provided for by way of meetings between the doctor, physiotherapist, occupational therapist, teacher, social workers, child psychologist, potential employer, the child and parents. Children of both sexes become much more conscious of the appearance of an artificial limb at puberty.

Those suffering from conditions such as spina bifida or arthrogryphosis, or who have experienced severe burns or trauma in childhood, may, after expert consultation and assessment, decide on amputation to improve function and cosmesis (see Ch. 20).

PRE-OPERATIVE PHYSIOTHERAPY

Physical assessment

The physiotherapist should start the pre-amputation assessment before the actual decision to amputate has been made if the status of the limb appears critical. The patient should be receiving treatment in a general surgical, medical, orthopaedic or plastic surgery ward and can be observed closely during this time. The possibility of amputation must not be divulged to the patient; this is solely the surgeon's responsibility.

The physiotherapist must read the patient's medical notes, drug chart and nursing records before planning the order of the initial assessment.

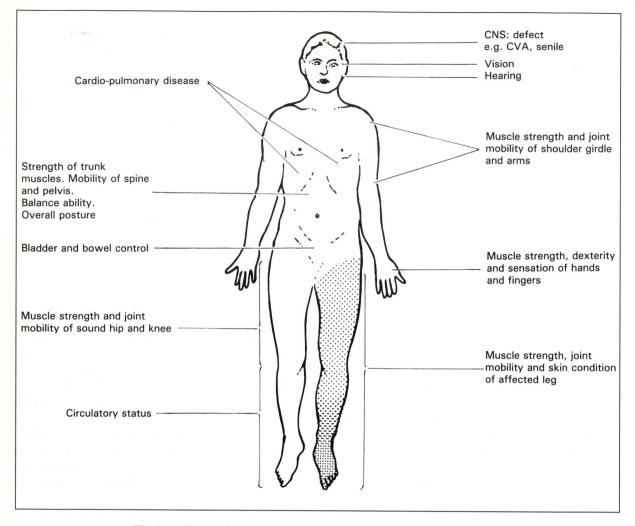

Fig. 2.2   Physical factors to be considered in the pre-amputation assessment.

The information to be gathered is as shown in Figure 2.2 and must be accurately recorded on either an assessment chart or treatment card.

Muscle strength, range of joint movement and functional mobility must be recorded so that future comparison is possible. When measuring a joint, a goniometer must be used. The hip should always be measured in Thomas' position (see Fig. 2.3). A number of positions can be used to measure the knee, but whatever method is chosen it is essential that subsequent readings are taken in the same position. The size and position of fragile pressure areas should also be accurately recorded.

It must be remembered, however, that assessment is on-going and never a 'one-off' exercise. Frequently the patient may be so systemically ill that accurate and detailed assessment is not possible. The physiotherapist and patient must gradually build up a relationship so that communication is free and detailed subjective information can be gathered. Many patients are confused, in pain and anxious at this time, and subjective information may be inaccurate at this stage. Therefore, whenever possible, the relatives or carers should be approached. The physical assessment and pre-operative exercise programme merge into being one and the same activity. The

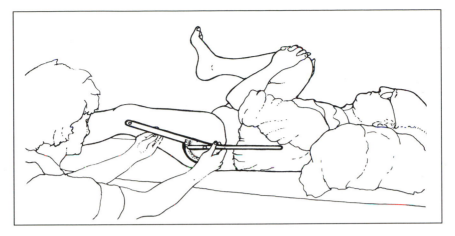

Fig. 2.3 Thomas' test for measurement of hip flexion contracture.

aims and goals of treatment should start to be planned at this stage.

Treating the patient in this situation will require a tactful approach, and care with the wording of questions is needed. The process of assessment must never cause the patient undue pain or distress — this will not build up confidence between the patient and physiotherapist. Timing physiotherapy sessions around analgesia is often essential for the best possible response. To eliminate repetition it may be possible for the physiotherapist to be present at the doctor's initial examination, or for the occupational therapist and physiotherapist to observe some activities together. It may be appropriate to contact self-help organisations, e.g. NALD, BLESMA, if the patient and/or relatives wish to discuss the future with another amputee.

Social assessment

Although the social assessment is not separate from the physical assessment, specific facts must be ascertained concerning the patient's home environment, support from relatives or friends, place and type of work, and the effect, if any, of the present medical condition on the patient's lifestyle. These questions can be asked during the physical assessment while the patient is resting between one activity and another, so that the sessions are not too tiring.

Frequently, it is the physiotherapist who sees the patient first, and from the initial assessment other members of the team can be alerted to specific problems requiring their special skills. It is essential that there is free and frequent communication between all members of the team to ensure that problems are clarified as soon as it is practicable.

It must also be remembered that the patient may relate a slightly different version of the situation to different team members and an accurate composite picture must be obtained by all.

Any services already being provided in the home should be known to the hospital team.

Pre-operative treatment

An active programme of pre-operative treatment may not be possible because of the medical condition of the patient, but the items listed below in the treatment plan should be attempted. Although the patient should ideally be brought to the physiotherapy department, this may not be possible if infection is present, drips are in situ, confusion is observed, or the patient is reluctant to be moved.

There will be many pre-operative investigations and assessments being carried out by the other team members and the relative importance of all aspects of pre-operative care must be recognised.

Treatment plan

a. *Pre-anaesthetic chest physiotherapy*. Many patients are smokers. Any postural drainage position can be used as necessary, provided that care is taken with the affected limb.

b. *Teach bed mobility*. A suitable high/low bed with a firm base, cot sides and a monkey pole should be provided pre-operatively so the patient can be taught bed mobility.

The patient having an upper limb amputation is shown how to move up and down the bed, and climb in and out of bed using one arm for support. The problems of balance postoperatively are explained to the patient.

The bed for the lower limb amputee must be adjustable so that the patient can transfer safely onto a wheelchair or commode. The firm base is necessary for balance. It must be explained to the patient that the cot sides are to aid mobility when rolling from side to side in the first few days postoperatively, and are not there because the staff expect the patient to be confused.

Use of the monkey pole for lifting up onto bedpans and relief of pressure areas is needed while the patient is relatively immobile. As the patient becomes stronger postoperatively, push-ups will be taught and the monkey pole will be taken away as soon as the patient can manage without it.

Observation of all areas of the skin is important as, particularly with negroid and Asian skin tones, erythema or ischaemic changes are harder to detect. Suitable care of pressure areas, particularly toes, heels, sacrum, trochanters and elbows, must be provided by the whole team.

c. *Teach transfers*. A standing pivot transfer using the unaffected leg is taught, but if the patient is unable to do this a sliding board may be used, or a backwards transfer if neither leg can bear weight (see Figs 3.8, 3.9, 3.10).

d. *Preserve joint mobility*. All joints must be treated. Active exercise is the ideal method of treatment. Passive stretching and positioning may be used.

If there is a slight contracture present in either a hip or knee joint, pre-operative treatment gives the best chance of regaining full range of movement. Postoperatively this becomes much harder,

not only because handling the limb produces more pain, but the lever arm is shorter. The prone position should only be used if the patient can tolerate it without respiratory distress or undue discomfort (see Ch. 3).

However, if there is a gross contracture present, which after a week's treatment has shown no sign of improvement, this must be reported to the surgeon as it may have direct bearing on the choice of level of amputation.

Full mobility of both shoulder joints and the shoulder girdle is essential for any level of upper limb amputation.

e. *Strengthen all muscles*. Upper limb, trunk and lower limb muscles must all be treated within the limits of the patient's tolerance; this may be only a few gentle bed exercises in the ward, or it may be a half hour programme in the treatment area.

f. *Teach wheelchair mobility*. The therapist should loan a suitable wheelchair pre-operatively. The patient is taught correct use of the brakes and foot plates (to ensure that damage does not occur to the skin of the lower legs) and how to manipulate the wheelchair (see Ch. 5).

g. *Walking wherever possible*. This is the best active exercise for preservation of muscle strength, joint mobility and function of the lower limbs. Memory of the gait pattern is maintained, even if only a few lengths of the parallel bars are

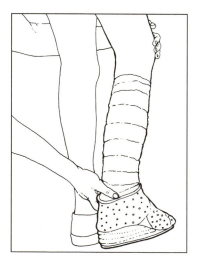

Fig. 2.4 Plastazote shoe, with a heel raise to encourage heel strike.

managed. However, it has been shown in one study at Queen Mary's University Hospital that only about 15% of patients can walk immediately prior to amputation of the lower limb. Plastazote shoes can be made to fit over dressings or bandages on the affected foot, thus relieving pressure. If there is a hip and/or knee flexion contracture, a heel raise will be necessary to obtain a positive heel strike, thus facilitating the extensor muscles (see Figs 2.4–2.7).

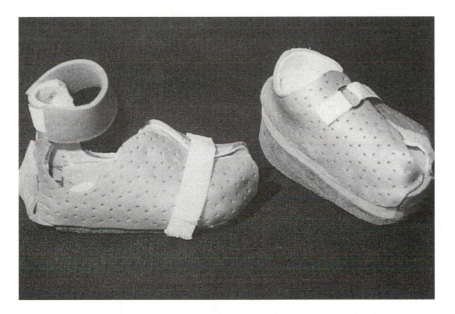

Fig. 2.5 Two designs of Plastazote shoe with Velcro fastenings and cork soles.

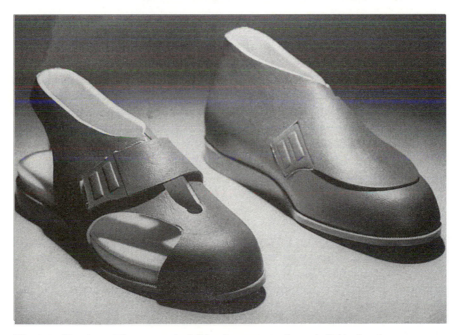

Fig. 2.6 Drushoes. The one on the left has been cut out for an individual patient. (Photograph by kind permission of John Drew (London) Ltd.)

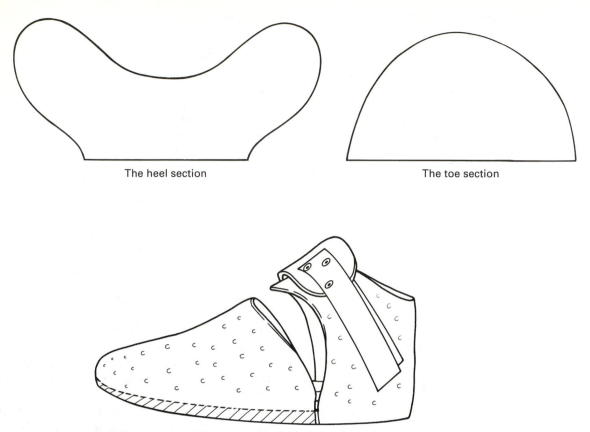

The heel section   The toe section

The completed Plastozote shoe with Velcro fastening

Fig. 2.7 The construction of a Plastazote shoe.

h. *Phantom sensation.* The patient is warned that it is completely normal to feel the sensation of the whole limb after amputation. This sensation gradually diminishes as active rehabilitation, including stump handling, resisted exercises and weightbearing, progresses, (see Ch. 19).

i. *Treatment for co-existing conditions.* Fractures, burns, backache, soft tissue lesions, etc. may also need specific treatment.

Both the patient and relatives should be made aware of the reasons, stages and timing involved in the rehabilitation process. The amount of detailed information given must be within the level of understanding of each person. This information may be given by the physiotherapist or another member of the team. As many relatives only visit at evenings and weekends, the nurse or doctor must be available then.

The physiotherapist must be very sensitive to the reactions of the patient at this stage as some denial of the situation may be present. However, practical queries may be better clarified, either for the patient or for the relatives or carers, by another amputee of similar age and with the same level of amputation. The opportunity to discuss social, economic, personal, domestic and mobility issues may allay fears more effectively than by lengthy discussion with the hospital staff.

Care must be taken if the patient wishes to see the type of prosthesis that they will use in the future. This is because the level of amputation may not have been finally decided and the type of prosthesis in the display cupboard of a general hospital may be old-fashioned and out of date.

DISCUSSION OF CHOICE OF AMPUTATION LEVEL

It is the responsibility of each team member to communicate their thoughts regarding the most desirable amputation level to the consultant surgeon. In making this decision the clinical, physical, social and psychological assessments will be taken into account, along with consideration of the prosthetic possibilities.

As amputation is a final decision, and as so many different professions are involved, a case conference may be the best setting for discussion to take place. This will naturally lead to a unified approach to the individual patient.

THE OVERALL CARE TEAM

1. *The physiotherapist*

The physiotherapist sees the patient throughout all stages of the rehabilitation programme, although more than one individual may be involved. Physiotherapists are the link members of the team overseeing and treating from pre- to postoperative stages, in pre- and postprosthetic mobility education and continuing with follow-up in the community throughout the patient's life. This will involve communication with the acute hospital, various out-patient and disablement services centre clinics, other hospitals, the community units and local authorities. Advice and support are also given regarding employment, sports and leisure activities.

2. *The surgeon*

The surgeon's role is to diagnose, order medical investigations, prescribe drugs and ultimately to inform the patient and relatives of the severity of the condition and necessity for amputation. Wherever possible amputations should be carried out in special units where consultant expertise is supported by the multidisciplinary team. Selection of level should be determined by team discussion and all should understand the implications of wearing a prosthesis. The rehabilitation consultant and prosthetist may be consulted prior to surgery. Postoperative medical treatment will be directed by the surgeon.

3. *The nurse*

The 24-hour observation of the patient is undertaken by the nurse who inevitably will take on a coordinating role. On admission an assessment is made of the patient's physical, psychological and social background, and an individual care plan is devised to take account of fluid balance and nutritional state; infection, pain, toxicity secondary to pain or infection; preservation of skin — especially sacrum, heels and elbows; spiritual and emotional needs; mobility.

Following surgery the care plan will include monitoring and relief of pain, daily observation and treatment of the stump and remaining leg, and emotional support regarding altered body image, lifestyle and reduced mobility. Supervision of other activities, e.g. transfers, exercises, etc, is carried out as a continuation of the treatment plans of other members of the multidisciplinary team, so communication between everyone is vital.

Involvement of the relatives and friends is vital from admission in order to promote an understanding of the aims of the many facets of care and rehabilitation. Liaison with other nursing colleagues already involved in the patient's care is maintained; this may include the health visitor, diabetic nurse specialist, district nurses, community psychiatric nurse and incontinence advisor. The hospital stay is only a transient phase of the patient's life and it is important that links with existing professional resources and those of family and friends are maintained in order to prevent a developing dependency need through the hospital stay.

The nurse is often the member of the team who explains and reassures both patients and relatives, and offers counselling and emotional support. Where appropriate the nurse will also encourage and supervise the patient in exercises and other techniques at week-ends and during evenings.

4. *The occupational therapist*

The occupational therapist's role is to enable the patient to return, where possible, to their previous lifestyle or to help them to reach their fullest potential within the limits of their disability. To this end information will be sought regarding their previous activities and home, and an opportunity will be given to discuss the patients hopes and expectations, fears and anxieties about the amputation and the future.

The OT may assess and supply the patient with a suitable wheelchair and cushion (although in some districts this may be done by the physiotherapist).

Assessment of activities of daily living will be carried out in the hospital and supply of specialised aids and adaptations will be carried out following assessment of the home, school or workplace and, after liaison with the local authority, other members of the household, or employers.

The prosthetic rehabilitation of the upper limb amputee is almost exclusively managed by the occupational therapist (see Ch. 17).

5. *The social worker*

The role of the social worker in the care of the amputee is to enable the therapeutic team to understand the patient and his needs more clearly. The objectives of early assessment are to ascertain some of the areas which may influence the treatment programme.

Ideally, the patient should be seen prior to amputation, although often, as in trauma cases, this is not possible. The two identifiable aims of assessment can broadly be seen as:

a. To help the patient and the family seek realistic solutions to any social or economic problems related to hospitalisation, and to the loss of a limb.
b. To help the patient and family express and understand the emotional reactions triggered off by amputation.

By understanding the patient and family, the team is better equipped to assess the patient's expectations and attitudes towards impending disability. Expectations will be built on the patient's personal life experience and previous ability to cope with both stress and possible hospital dependency.

During the initial stages the patient will have to rely on both old and new-found experiences and

psychological resources. The extent to which patients are understood by the team will directly affect their reactions whilst they are undergoing treatment and restructuring their lives. The foundation of building up a relationship with the patient in the early days will undoubtedly be beneficial to all concerned. It must be said that the individual patient will generally choose the staff member in whom they will confide and therefore all members of the team should be prepared to fulfil a supporting role.

For many patients, the aura of hospital, white coats and uniforms may be bewildering. Often they cannot comprehend the necessity for extreme surgical action. For instance, they may not see immediately the justification for amputating a gangrenous toe or foot, or badly fractured ankle with vascular involvement; therefore, explanation in simple non-medical terms is needed. The medical implications of the treatment and prognosis should also be explained to the family, for they are often the mainstay of support in and out of hospital. It is hoped that by this full explanation any rejection of the patient for being a burden to the family will be avoided.

Gradual preparation is essential. In some cases the possibility of impending bereavement must be faced by the family, and help should be given to them in coping with their emotions and the practical arrangements that have to be made.

It is often assumed that the elderly have more problems than the younger amputee, but this is not so. Obviously the younger amputee is usually fitter, healthier and more agile at the time of amputation; the problems are different, but no less important.

The elderly patient. Major surgery such as amputation may well exacerbate the ageing process. Understanding the individual's attitude and outlook prior to amputation may give the therapeutic team some insight into how the patient will cope with a profound change. Housing may be an immediate problem, and this will require early assessment and action. Any delay in this procedure could lead to prolonged hospitalisation for the patient and may cause a deterioration in the rehabilitation process. If initial information gained gives rise for concern, then an early home visit in conjunction with the family, social worker, occupational therapist and physiotherapist should be made.

The relevant legislation for the disabled is the Chronically Sick and Disabled Persons Act 1970 Section 2, and The Disabled Persons (Services, Consultation and Representation) Act 1986 Section 4. These sections confirm that a local authority must assess the needs of a disabled person for any service listed in Section 2 of the Chronically Sick and Disabled Persons Act 1970 if asked to do so by the disabled person, authorised person or carer. The 1970 Act requires social services departments to make arrangements for the provisions of a variety of services if they are satisfied that they are needed by anyone who is permanently and substantially handicapped. The services listed are help in the home, recreational facilities in the home, recreational facilities outside the home (daycare), transport, aids and adaptations, holiday, meals and telephones.

Local authorities are obliged to seek suitable housing for the disabled person. However, in certain parts of the UK there is an acute shortage of such housing and although pressure brought to bear on the relevant housing department will eventually bring results it is a process that should be approached with vigour and energy.

For the younger amputee, school or employment may have to be modified or changed radically, depending on the amputee's potential for rehabilitation. These negotiations may be undertaken directly with the employers or help may be sought from the community disablement resettlement officers attached to most job centres. The underlying fears of discontinued employment may often go undetected in the initial stages but should be investigated at the earliest opportunity, so that the patient can be given something to work towards.

For all amputees, financial worries can affect the family as well as the patient. There are various benefits which can be applied for; information can be obtained from DSS offices, or from hospital or community social services departments. The most relevant benefit for the amputee is the mobility allowance; this is a controversial benefit and is often refused following the first application. An appeal against the decision is often worthwhile and successful.

The need for communication during the initial stages between all members of the therapeutic team is strongly indicated; good communication gives the best chance to the patient and therapist for successful rehabilitation.

The changes brought about by the Care in the Community Act of Parliament will inevitably have implications for the amputee and his carers once discharged home. The team looking after the patient in hospital must be aware of procedures with their local authority and ensure that a needs assessment is carried out as early as possible.

6. *The consultant in rehabilitation*

The rehabilitation consultant's role is to provide long-term, committed medical leadership for the needs of the amputee throughout his or her life. In the pre-operative assessment phase, the rehabilitation physician will advise the surgeon on the optimal level and technique of amputation in difficult cases.

In the immediate postoperative phase a disability-orientated, holistic assessment is carried out, considering co-existing pathologies, psychological and social problems. A realistic appraisal of the future outcome of rehabilitation is discussed with the multidisciplinary team, patient and carers, and a proposed plan is made. The prescription for the first prosthesis is made and the physician will ensure early monitoring of both the stump and the prognosis of the general condition of the patient.

In the follow-up phase, reappraisal of the patient's progress is made and refinement of the prosthetic prescription carried out as functional ability changes. Maintenance of the prosthesis and updating are carried out as monitoring of the changing needs of the patient and advancement in hardwear supply indicate. It is often later, i.e. about 1 year following discharge from hospital, that the leisure needs and sports activities of the patient need careful prosthetic reassessment to optimise performance. The rehabilitation physician will also identify and treat problems such as stump skin complications, phantom and stump pain, and will consult other specialists as necessary. Links with staff in the community are made, e.g. GP, physiotherapist, occupational therapist, nurse, etc, to ensure the coordinated and specialised aftercare of the amputee.

A research role is expected by means of clinical audit, evaluation of resource use and original clinical research; the rehabilitation consultant will also have a teaching role with junior medical staff and students, as well as with other members of the multidisciplinary team.

7. *The prosthetist*

The prosthetist's role is to provide care to patients with partial or total absence of a limb by designing, fabricating and fitting a prosthesis (artificial limb).

The prosthetist is responsible for understanding and specifying the limb design, selecting materials and components, making all necessary casts, measurements and model modifications, including static and dynamic alignments. The prosthetist will evaluate the prosthesis on the patient, give instructions in its use, refer on to a physiotherapist or occupational therapist for further training, and maintain patient records. In consultation with the referring doctor, the prosthetist may formulate the prescription for the limb following examination and evaluation of the patient's prosthetic needs.

Additionally, the prosthetist is expected to keep abreast of new developments and to supervise the functions of support personnel and laboratory activities related to the production and development of the prostheses.

The prosthetist will remain the contact point for all the prosthetic needs of the amputee throughout their limb-wearing life. New prostheses and designs can be advised on and amputees can be put in touch with each other through the prosthetist regarding leisure and sports activities.

REFERENCES

Barsby P, Lumley J S P 1987 Check-list for the management of the lower limb amputee. Surgery 41: 985–986

Bradway J K, Malone J M, Racy J, Leal J M, Poole J 1984 Psychological adaptation to amputation: an overview. Orthotics and Prosthetics 38(3): 46–50

Bruce J 1991 The function and operation of a parent support association. Prosthetics and Orthotics International 15: 160–161

Clifford P C, Davies P W, Hayne J A, Baird R N 1980 Intermittent claudication: is a supervised exercise class worthwhile? British Medical Journal 21 June: 1503–1505

Crowther H 1982 New perspectives on nursing lower limb amputees. Journal of Advanced Nursing 7: 453–460

Day H J B 1979 Congenital lower limb deformities and extension prostheses. Physiotherapy 65(1): 3

Day H J B 1991 The ISO/ISPO classification of congenital limb deficiency. Prosthetics and Orthotics International 15: 67–69

Dean E 1987 Assessment of the peripheral circulation: an update for practitioners. The Australian Journal of Physiotherapy 33(3): 164–171

Dowd G S E, Linge K, Bentley G 1983 Measurement of transcutaneous oxygen pressure in normal and ischaemic skin. Journal of Bone and Joint Surgery 65-B(1): 79–83

Earl H M, Souhami R L 1990 Adolescent bone tumours: osteosarcomas and Ewing's sarcomas. The Practitioner 234: 816–818

English A W G 1989 Psychology of limb loss. British Medical Journal 299 : 1287

Evans D G R, Thakker Y, Donnai D 1991 Heredity and dysmorphic syndromes in congenital limb deficiencies. Prosthetics and Orthotics International 15: 70–77

Falkel J E 1983 Amputation as a consequence of diabetes mellitus. Physical Therapy 63(6): 960–964

Fyfe N C M 1990 An audit of amputation levels in patients referred for prosthetic rehabilitation. Prosthetics and Orthotics International 14: 67–70

Ham R O, Van de Ven C 1991 Patterns of recovery for lower limb amputation in the UK. WCPT 11th International Congress Proceedings Book II, p 658–660

Holstein P 1982 Level selection in leg amputation for arterial occlusive disease. Acta Orthopaedica Scandinavica 53: 821–831

Hunter J, Middleton F R I 1984 Cold injury amputees — a psychosocial problem? Prosthetics and Orthotics International 8: 143–146

Jackson J 1989 The role of the counsellor with amputees. Step Forward 16 (Autumn)

Jacobs P A 1984 Limb salvage and rotationplasty for osteosarcoma in children. Clinical Orthopaedics and Related Research 188: 217–222

Jamieson C W, Hill D 1976 Amputation for vascular disease. British Journal of Surgery 63: 683–690

Kasabian A K, Colen S R, Shaw W W, Pachter H L 1991 The role of microvascular free flaps in salvaging below-knee amputation stumps: a review of 22 cases. Journal of Trauma 31(4): 495–501

Krebs D E, Edelstein J E, Thornby M A 1991 Prosthetic management of children with limb deficiencies. Physical Therapy 71(12): 920–934

Lange L R 1982 Prosthetic implications with the diabetic patient. Orthotics and Prosthetics 36(2): 96–102

Lempberg R, Ahlgren O 1982 Prosthetic replacement of tumour-destroyed diaphyseal bone in the lower extremity. Acta Orthopaedica Scandinavica 53: 541–545

Liedberg E, Persson B M 1983 Age, diabetes and smoking in lower limb amputation for arterial occlusive disease. Acta Orthopaedica Scandinavica 54: 383–388

Lind J, Kramhoft M, Bodtker 1991 The influence of smoking on complications after amputations of the lower extremity. Clinical Orthopaedics and Related Research 267 (June 91): 211–217

Murray Parkes C 1972 Components of the reaction to loss of a limb, spouse or home. Journal of Psychosomatic Research 16: 343–349

Murray Parkes C, Napier M M 1970 Psychiatric sequelae of amputation. British Journal of Hospital Medicine 4(5): 610–614

O'Riordain D S, O'Donnell J A 1991 Realistic expectations for the patient with intermittent claudication. British Journal of Surgery 78: 861–863

Reardon J A, Curwen I H M, Jarman P, Dewar M, Chodera J 1982 Thermography and leg ulceration. Acta Thermographica 7(1): 18–23

Redhead R G 1984 The place of amputation in the management of the ischaemic lower limb in the dysvascular geriatric patient. International Rehabilitation Medicine 6: 68–71

Roberts A 1988 Systems of life No. 160. Senior systems – 25. Peripheral vascular disease – 1. Nursing Times 84(18): 49–52

Rose C A H, McIntosh C S 1991 Diabetes in the limb fitting centre. Practical Diabetes 8(4): 146–147

Scales J T 1983 Bone and joint replacement for the preservation of limbs. British Journal of Hospital Medicine 30: 220–232

Setoguchi Y 1991 The management of the limb deficient child and its family. Prosthetics and Orthotics International 15: 78–81

Simon M A, Aschliman M A, Thomas N 1986 Limb-salvage treatment versus amputation for osteosarcoma of the distal end of the femur. Journal of Bone and Joint Surgery 68A(9): 1331–1337

Spence V A, Walker W F, Troup I M, Murdoch G 1981 Amputation of the ischaemic limb: selection of the optimum site by thermography. Angiology 32: 155–169

Spence V A, McCollum P T, Walker W F, Murdoch G 1984 Assessment of tissue viability in relation to the selection of amputation level. Prosthetics and Orthotics International 8: 67–75

Sweetman R 1980 Tumours of bone and their treatment today. British Journal of Hospital Medicine 24(5): 452–463

Torode I P, Gillespie R 1991 The classification and treatment of proximal femoral deficiencies. Prosthetics and Orthotics International 15: 117–126

Wake P, Mansfield A O 1980 Vascular surgery of the lower limb. British Journal of Hospital Medicine Aug: 120–129

Williams L R et al 1991 Vascular rehabilitation: benefits of a structured exercise/risk modification programme. Journal of Vascular Surgery 14: 320–326

3. Early postoperative treatment

The care and treatment given to the amputee at the early postoperative stage is concerned with mobility both in bed and about the immediate surroundings of the ward. It commences on the first postoperative day and is continued for as long as the patient's condition indicates.

For the younger patient who is physically fit and has normal vascularity, the prime consideration is healing of the wound. The wound drains may remain in situ for a few days and movement may therefore be restricted. Prevention of contractures and wound management are the most important factors at this time. It may be unnecessary to give general mobilising and strengthening exercises to these patients in the first 2–3 postoperative days.

In contrast, the patient suffering from vascular disease and diabetes is generally older, unfit and possibly confused, and is thus more at risk from the complications of bed rest, i.e. bronchopneumonia, pressure sores, urinary tract infection, etc. Therefore, immediate mobilisation on the first or second postoperative day is recommended.

Chest care is started immediately but other exercises are added as the patient responds. Postoperatively, all amputees experience a certain amount of pain, and this must be adequately controlled, particularly during the very early stages. Physiotherapy must be organised around analgesia; short but frequent treatments given daily achieve the best result.

The correct bed and accessories should have been organised pre-operatively (see Ch. 2, p. 14). The type of mattress, sheets and other pressure care items must also be considered, particularly as in the first 2–3 postoperative days the patient finds alternate side lying uncomfortable for long periods. It may be necessary to add sheepskins, foam pads, sponge leg gutters, etc., to protect the remaining foot and leg. Bed cradles are necessary to relieve pressure of bedclothes from the stump and dorsum of the remaining foot.

PHYSIOTHERAPY

Following amputation, the patient may have difficulty in coming to terms with the stump psychologically as it is sometimes very unsightly during the initial stages of healing. Some patients may not look at the stump for some time and may deny to themselves that amputation has been performed. For others it may be a very gradual process of acceptance. It has been noted that if the entire therapeutic staff refer to and handle the stump normally, then the patient can learn to accept this new concept of his body. If this fails, then there are a few who will present with the syndrome of distorted body image. Gentle acknowledgement of reality and reinforcement will help this type of patient make this major physical and psychological adjustment. However, there are a few patients who never fully achieve this.

It is important that the physiotherapist, at the first postoperative treatment session, observes the patient's ability to move the stump independently. Handling the stump should first be attempted by the patient, before the physiotherapist provides either assistance or resistance to movement. Sensitivity of approach is necessary at this first session, as it may be the first time the patient touches the stump and fully realises that amputation has taken place.

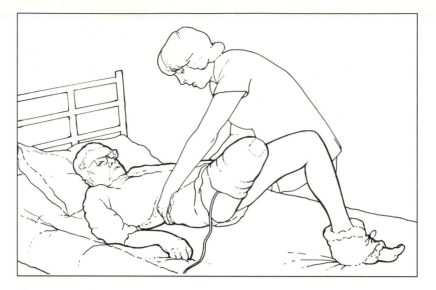

Fig. 3.1   An above-knee amputee bridging on the first postoperative day.

Active movements

The active movements which are attempted first are hip flexion, extension, adduction and abduction, static quadriceps and knee flexion exercises, and contractions of the muscles in the below-knee stump. To aid bed mobility, exercises such as bridging, rolling, moving up and down the bed, sitting forwards and pushing up using the arms, can be attempted on the first postoperative day and continued until the patient is fully mobile in bed. Active exercise of the remaining limb can also lead to 'overflow' to the stump, thus encouraging active movement.

All these techniques, except push-ups, can be attempted with drips, drains or catheters in situ (see Figs 3.1–3.3). The physiotherapist should continue to encourage the patient to gently touch the stump over the dressings, to assist movement, re-educate sensation and aid psychological acceptance. Vascular and diabetic patients must always take great care when moving about so that neither the stump nor the remaining leg is

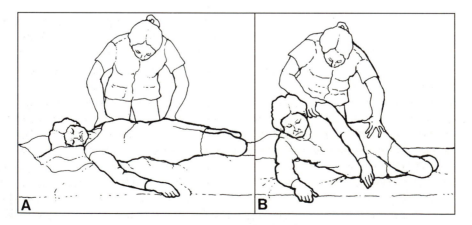

Fig. 3.2   A bilateral below-knee amputee rolling. Note the hand positions of the physiotherapist.

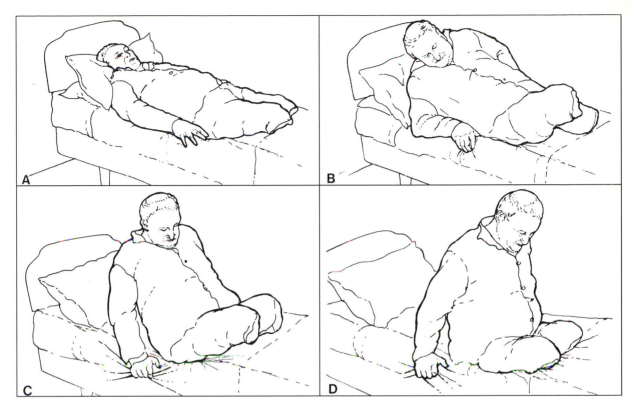

Fig. 3.3 A bilateral above-knee amputee sitting up in bed. Note arm positions and trunk rotation.

knocked on the cot sides or the bed cradle. Even this minor trauma can cause a major complication; any team member who observes this must report to the doctor immediately. It is more difficult to observe minor damage to the skin of negroid or Asian patients, so the team must be constantly vigilant.

Prevention of contractures

1. If the amputation is below the knee joint, the knee must rest in full extension immediately after the operation. Any dressing applied should not pull the stump into flexion. Pain frequently causes a flexor withdrawal pattern, involving both hip and knee, and must not be allowed to persist; sufficient analgesia must therefore to given.

The physiotherapist can passively extend a below-knee stump, temporarily fixed in flexion, after a night's sleep or a midday rest, by placing both hands either side of the knee, pushing the patella proximally with the thumbs and sliding

the tibia forwards with the fingers (Fig. 3.4). Once full extension has been achieved the patient is able to perform static quadriceps exercises and maintain the extended position independently. This extended position is maintained by providing a stump board for the wheelchair (Figs 3.5 and 3.6).

The use of weights, sandbags and pillows to maintain this position is inadvisable. The weight of these objects can occlude circulation in the stump which causes pain, which in turn causes increased flexor withdrawal.

2. If the amputation is through or above the knee joint the major concern is the development of a hip flexion contracture, but it must be remembered that the short above-knee stump can also become abducted as a result of the un-opposed pull of the intact gluteus medius and gluteus minimus. Active hip extension and adduction exercises must be given. However, the long above-knee and through-knee stumps can become adducted because the strong pull of the

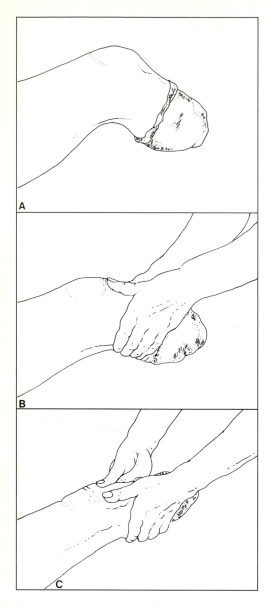

Fig. 3.4 Passive extension of a below-knee stump.

long intact adductor longus and adductor brevis is greater than that of the hip abductors. Therefore, in these cases active hip extension and abduction exercises must be given.

3. The patient will, of necessity, be sitting up in bed or in the wheelchair for long periods of time. Therefore, set periods of either supine or prone lying, to obtain neutral hip alignment,

must become part of the daily routine. Although the prone lying position is the most effective, it is not usually tolerated by the patient in the immediate postoperative period. Some patients with cardiorespiratory problems, kyphotic spine or gross arthritis will never achieve this position comfortably, and so should not be expected to do so.

The treatment programme must be gradually altered each day to attain the correct positioning; i.e. supine lying for only 10 minutes may be all that is possible for some patients; others will progress to prone lying for $\frac{1}{2}$ hour, twice a day (see Fig. 3.7).

4. All joints in the upper and lower limbs and trunk must be actively treated, as contractures and loss of range of movement of any joint can occur while the patient is relatively immobile.

Transfers

The stage at which patients are able to sit out of bed in a wheelchair will be governed by their medical condition. The general rule is that the patient must be alert and capable of responding to instruction. It is often the physiotherapist's responsibility to decide when the patient is capable of this response, the method of transfer most suitable, and to give both instruction and help with the transfer. It is possible to transfer the patient into the wheelchair while the drip, wound drain and catheter are still in situ if suitable care is taken, which may be as early as the first or second postoperative day.

A suitable wheelchair should have been loaned pre-operatively and must be self-propelling (see Ch. 2); the amputee should not sit in a static armchair. The use of the wheelchair greatly improves both the physical and psychological state of the patient. The assessment for a suitable and safe loan wheelchair must be carried out by a qualified therapist, who will also decide on the need for, and prescription of, a permanent wheelchair (see Ch. 5).

Methods of transfer

The patient must have a well-fitting shoe on the

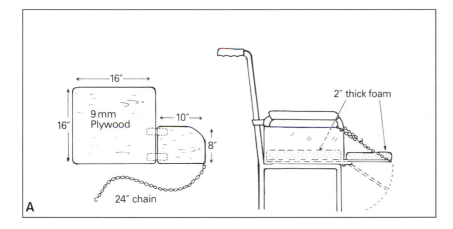

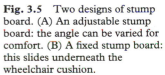

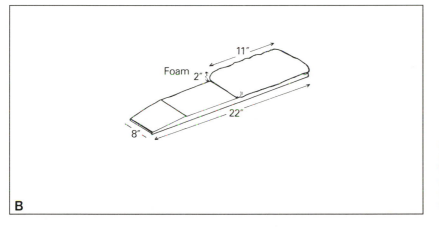

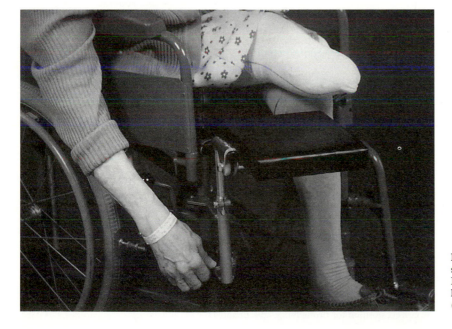

Fig. 3.5 Two designs of stump board. (A) An adjustable stump board: the angle can be varied for comfort. (B) A fixed stump board: this slides underneath the wheelchair cushion.

Fig. 3.6 The King's amputee stump board Mark II (made by Remploy Ltd). It is made in two lengths: medium (8 in) and long (11 in).

No pillows or *one* pillow

Arms positioned wherever comfortable for patient

Stump lying flat (with knee straight if b/k) *no pillow*

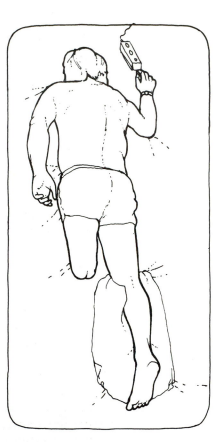

Nurse call bell placed within patient's reach

Head turned to sound side

Patient wearing a watch to time period prone

Both hips completely flat on bed

Remaining leg supported on a pillow to prevent toes from digging into bed

Footboard and bedclothes turned right back out of the way

POINTS TO REMEMBER
1. To roll prone, the patient must turn towards the sound side, the nurse ensuring that the stump is lowered gently.
2. Initially the patient lies prone for about 10 minutes.
3. The patient should then build up to lying prone for $\frac{1}{2}$ hour three times a day.

Fig. 3.7   The correct position for prone lying. (b/k denotes below-knee.)

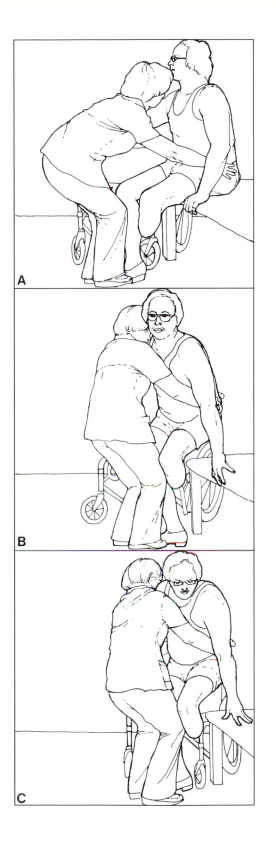

remaining foot before attempting to transfer. There are three methods of transfer for the amputee:

— Standing pivot transfer (Fig. 3.8)
— Backwards/forwards transfer (Fig. 3.9)
— Sliding board transfer (Fig. 3.10).

Once a safe method of transfer has been decided, the whole care team must be informed, so that the same method is always used and the patient is encouraged towards independence.

Use of the wheelchair (see Ch. 5)

After the method of transfer has been established, the patient must be taught how to manoeuvre the wheelchair safely. The brakes and footrests must be explained, demonstrated and fully understood by the patient and any attendant assisting. It is so easy to forget to apply the brakes when the wheelchair is stationary, or to knock the remaining leg with the foot rest. Detachable arm rests must be completely secure. A stump board must be provided for through-knee and below-knee stumps. This will protect the stump from knocks, prevent knee joint contracture and control oedema (Fig. 3.5, p. 27). Some patients with poor sitting balance, e.g. hemiplegics and bilateral amputees, may need a seat belt.

Patients with poor eyesight, hearing, weak hands or arms, and poor sensation, require lengthy instruction and practice in wheelchair management. The confused patient also requires constant supervision.

Young, fit and agile patients may be unwilling to use a wheelchair. The physiotherapist must explain the dangers of the dependent position of the stump while using crutches in these very early postoperative days. The problems of pain, oedema and the possibility of delayed wound healing must be understood by the younger patient.

Fig. 3.8 The standing pivot transfer. Note that (A) the wheelchair is at 45° to the bed, (B) the physiotherapists hands on the patient's pelvis and (C) her knees are blocking the knee of the patient's remaining leg.

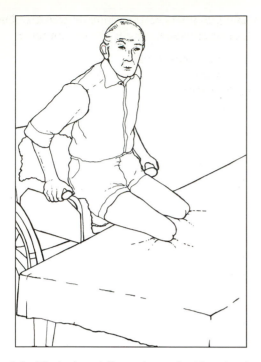

Fig. 3.9 The backwards/forwards transfer. Note that the wheelchair and bed are level. While this transfer is more often used by bilateral amputees, it is also suitable for other patients unable to bear weight on either leg.

Dressing practice

The patient should be up and dressed each day, before progression to treatment in the physiotherapy department can take place (see Ch. 4). However, if the patient requires help from the nurses to dress, the occupational therapist should start dressing practice in the ward when sitting balance has been achieved (Fig. 3.11). Most elderly patients need help or guidance, particularly with trousers and underpants. The hemiplegic or bilateral lower limb amputee, and the upper limb amputee, may need special dressing aids or adaptations.

Many patients find dressing very tiring, but should be encouraged to do as much as possible for themselves, and then be allowed to rest before carrying out strenuous exercise in the treatment areas.

It is important to note that if it is still impossible for a patient to put on underpants or trousers independently after daily dressing practice with the occupational therapist, it is very unlikely that the independent application of a prosthesis will be possible (see Ch. 6).

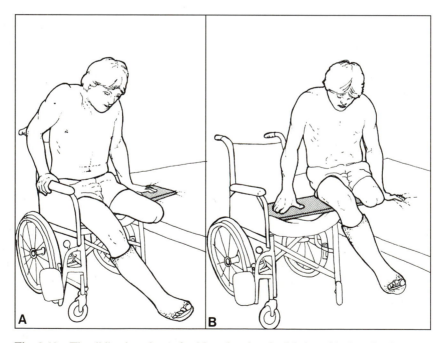

Fig. 3.10 The sliding board transfer. Note that the wheelchair and bed are level and that the sliding board is sufficiently long to allow the patient to slide smoothly over the gap between the bed and chair. This method is also ideal for transferring from wheelchair to car seat.

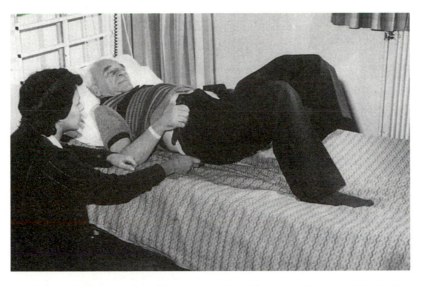

Fig. 3.11   Dressing practice with the occupational therapist. (Reproduced by kind permission of Faber & Faber, from Downie P A (ed) 1990 Cash's textbook of general medical and surgical conditions for physiotherapists.)

STUMP OEDEMA

Stump oedema occurs immediately after the operation as a result of surgical trauma and may also recur at any future time in the amputee's life from a variety of other causes (see Fig. 3.12). It is important that the physiotherapist recognises the total problem and all aspects of its management, so that the amputees can be taught to recognise it and thus cope with their own future management.

Methods of treatment of stump oedema

1. Elevation

The foot of the bed can be elevated, providing the blood pressure is stable and the vascularity of the stump and the remaining leg is adequate. The below-knee stump should be elevated on a stump board when using the wheelchair (see Fig. 3.6, p. 27). After discharge home, the patient can elevate the stump on a stool or chair.

2. Exercise

Active contraction of the stump muscles is the best method of reducing oedema. A regular

pumping action by the opposing muscle groups is needed.

— The below-knee amputee must imagine the performance of alternate dorsiflexion and plantar flexion in order to achieve this muscle contraction.
— The through-knee and above-knee amputee must perform alternate hip flexion and extension and hip abduction and adduction.

These active exercises must be performed at regular intervals throughout the day; 10 repetitions performed hourly is a useful guideline. Bilateral activities often achieve a more vigorous contraction in the amputated side. Any amputee who has strong and well coordinated stump muscles can look forward to a better prosthetic future, e.g. a strong and muscular above-knee stump is suitable for retaining a self-suspending socket and controlling a free-knee joint mechanism (see Ch. 11).

3. Bandaging

Bandaging should only be used to control oedema; it is a misconception to think that ban-

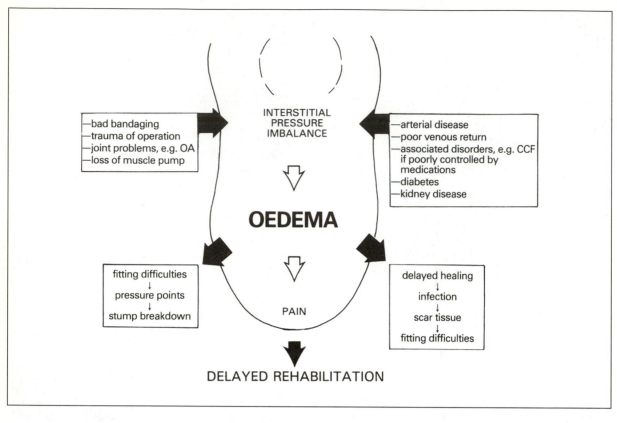

Fig. 3.12 Causes of stump oedema.

daging will shape the stump. Stump bandaging is a technique which has been used from the early 1900s. In those days the main reason for amputation was trauma and the majority of patients had normal stump vascularity. The prostheses then had simple conical-shaped sockets fashioned out of wood, and bandaging was important to enable the stump to fit into the socket. Today the considerations are very different.

a. Over 80% of new amputees now suffer from peripheral vascular disease and/or diabetes. The pressure exerted by a stump bandage can frequently exceed the arterial pressure in the blood vessels of the stump, causing pressure necrosis, which in turn can lead to a higher level of amputation. This is particularly true in the below-knee amputation. It is safer to dress the stump with just a light covering, e.g. Tubifast.

b. Surgeons are now fashioning the muscle flaps of the stump with greater expertise. This factor alone will determine the final shape of the stump: stump bandaging can never change stump shape without the danger of interference with the local circulation. Incorrect bandaging can, however, distort the tissues.

c. Prosthetists now have many more techniques and materials available for making the socket of the artificial limb fit the individual stump. It should be remembered that a uniformly oedematous stump is more readily fitted than one which has become misshapen with bandaging (see Fig. 3.13).

Bandaging may be required for tissue support and comfort, particularly for the young trauma amputee, who will contract the muscles against the support of the bandage. Then a crepe

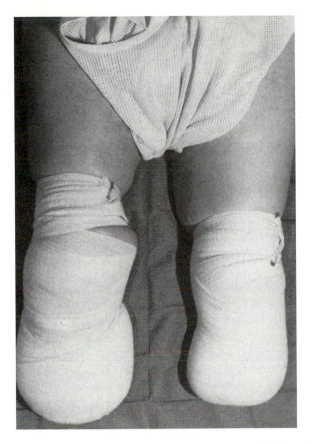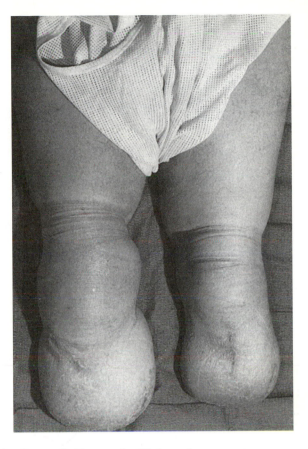

Fig. 3.13 The disastrous effect of bad bandaging: (A) shows the bandage applied incorrectly; (B) shows the uneven stump produced.

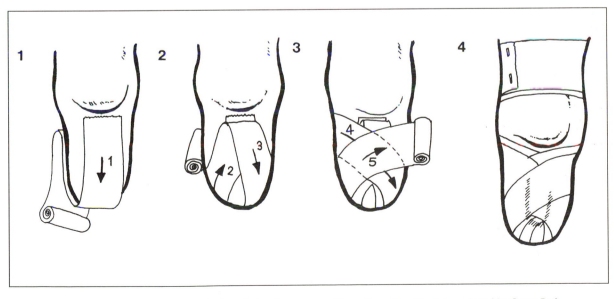

Fig. 3.14 The method of bandaging a below-knee stump. From the original leaflet produced by Seton Ltd.

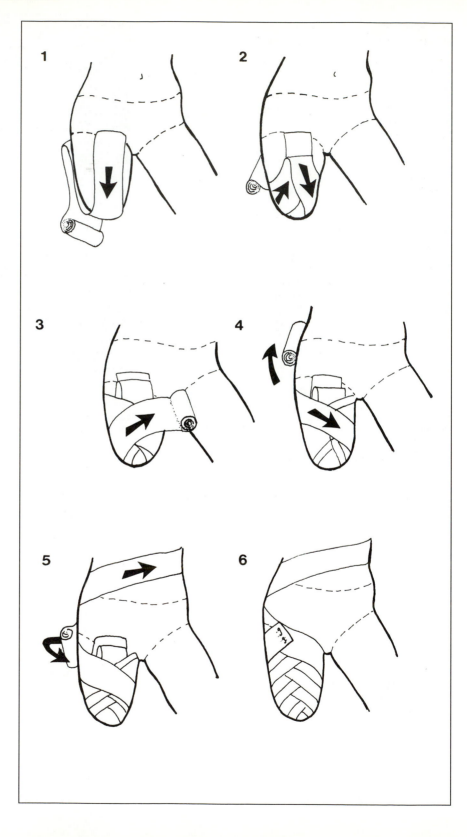

Fig. 3.15 The method of bandaging an above-knee stump. (From the original leaflet produced by Seton Ltd.)

bandage should be used prior to the removal of sutures from the wound, and a rayon and elastic bandage (e.g. Elset 'S') afterwards. Very few patients can apply the bandage themselves, but they should be absolutely familiar with the method and principles of bandaging (see Figs 3.14 and 3.15). The relatives or carers should be taught how to apply the bandage.

4. Intermittent variable air pressure machines (e.g. Flowtron)

There are a variety of these machines available, but the general principle employed is that, by varying the air pressure around the stump in a predetermined cyclic fashion, the circulation of blood and lymph can be modified with beneficial results. The pressures imposed by these machines on the tissues are uniform throughout the length of the stump, regardless of size or shape, so a tourniquet effect is impossible.

5. Pneumatic pylon

This pneumatic postamputation mobility aid (Ppam-Aid) can be used before prosthetic delivery, or for periods when the prosthesis no longer fits when oedema is present (for further description see Ch. 5).

Methods 1–5 can be used either separately or in combination, at either the early postoperative stage or at the prosthetic re-education stage, when the prosthesis supplied does not fit because of oedema (see Ch. 13).

6. Rigid dressing

Some young traumatic below-knee amputees may have a plaster-of-Paris dressing applied.

Plaster-of-Paris or other rigid material should not be used for any stump in which wound healing is doubtful. However, it can be very useful in specialised centres, where early postoperative temporary sockets made of either plaster-of-Paris or thermoplastic material, e.g. Hexalite, can be constructed. Early gait rehabilitation is then achieved.

7. Shrinker socks (e.g. Juzo)

These elasticated stump socks are available in various sizes from the DSC stores. They are only to be used for the healed stump with oedema. They are less likely to wrinkle and cause a tourniquet effect than other elasticated materials, as the correct size can be supplied. It is advisable that when the elasticated sock is first tried, it is worn for at least half an hour under the supervision of the physiotherapist. The stump must be observed carefully during this time for colour change and indentation, which may indicate that the sock is not the correct size. The sock should only be used when the patient is awake but not wearing the prosthesis, i.e. first thing in the morning when the patient gets out of bed and before the prosthesis is applied, and in the evening when the prosthesis is removed while the patient is sitting down. It is inadvisable to sleep wearing the elasticated sock, as damage to the stump may occur.

REFERENCES

Ham R, Richardson P 1986 The King's amputee stump board Mark II. Physiotherapy 72(3): 124

Hamilton A 1977 Device for supporting the stump of a below-knee amputee. Physiotherapy 63(10): 318

Koerner I 1976 To bandage or not to bandage: that is the question. Physiotherapy Canada 28(2): 75–78

Murdoch G 1983 The postoperative environment of the amputation stump. Prosthetics and Orthotics International 7: 75–78

Redhead R G, Snowdon C 1978 A new approach to the management of wounds of the extremities. Controlled environment treatment and its derivatives. Prosthetics and Orthotics International 2: 148–156

Sarmiento A 1972 Postoperative management. Orthopedic Clinics of North America 3(2): 435–446

Tilbury B, Slack H N, Mancey C 1985 The Exeter amputee stump support board. Physiotherapy 71(11): 477

4. Exercise programme

This chapter sets out the general fitness programme that is required for all ages and types of lower limb amputee. The treatment of the upper limb amputee is continued in Chapter 17. The exercises described may be carried out during all stages of progress, from about 1 week post-operatively up to and after the delivery of the prosthesis.

Illustrated here are examples and ideas for treatment, but every patient must be separately assessed and an appropriate scheme devised. This is a programme of general exercise which may be carried out in any department, large or small, or alternatively in the home.

THE NEW AMPUTEE

Following removal of the wound drain, the patient should be up and dressed during the day; the exercise programme can then continue in the physiotherapy department. For this programme to take place, it is necessary that the patient is not confused, the pain is adequately controlled and the patient's medical condition has stabilised (particularly important for diabetics). Incontinence should not prevent treatment, as catheters or tubing can be connected to a leg bag worn under the clothing, and special incontinence pads and pants are available. Exercises should be performed daily until delivery of the prosthesis.

It is ideal for patients to remain in hospital until they are fully rehabilitated on their prosthesis. Unfortunately, many hospitals discharge their patients after wound healing is complete and rehabilitation is still in its infancy. In the latter case, it is imperative that the patient attends for out-patient physiotherapy regularly, or is seen in the home by the community physiotherapist. It is most important that however difficult these arrangements are to make, the patient continues with an exercise regime until prosthetic re-education starts. Contractures, weakness and loss of function are often the result of inadequate supervision during this time. It is the hospital physiotherapist's responsibility to oversee the management of patients until they are fully rehabilitated and are using the prosthesis. This is not easy and much time and energy is required to ensure that the patient progresses smoothly through prosthetic fitting stages, and eventually achieves full prosthetic rehabilitation.

Those patients who are not progressing to prosthetic rehabilitation must also perform a daily exercise programme. As high a level of physical fitness, stamina and independence as possible must be obtained before the patient is discharged home using a wheelchair.

THE ESTABLISHED AMPUTEE PRESENTING WITH A NEW PROBLEM

If for any reason an established limb wearer cannot wear the prosthesis, the same principle of daily exercise must be followed. Examples of problems these patients may encounter are:

a. Stump breakdown
b. Surgical retrim of the stump
c. Other surgery, fracture or acute episode
d. Recurrence of tumour
e. Other medical conditions, e.g. minor stroke, diabetic upset, cardiorespiratory problems

f. Social difficulties.

If surgical revision to a higher level of amputation is carried out, the patient must be regarded as a new amputee. Balance, proprioception and muscle control are altered and the patient must realise that using the new prosthesis will be very different. The full exercise programme must be given.

AIMS OF TREATMENT RELATED TO AGE

The aims of rehabilitation are basically the same for all age groups, namely personal, domestic, social and economic competence. There are, however, specific factors to be taken into account when planning treatment programmes, always bearing in mind each individual's needs.

The young. The aims of the physical treatment for the young are perfection of movement, co-ordination and full muscle strength. These patients become easily bored, so that constant variation and imagination in their exercise programme is necessary. Realistically hard exercises must be given with daily progression, with particular emphasis on the stump. The physiotherapist must also be prepared to give time and find the opportunity to listen carefully to the younger amputee and maybe to prompt them, in a sensitive manner, into voicing their concerns. Often these patients are discharged home from hospital quickly and by the time they have found out what is involved in their changed circumstances, opportunities for receiving information and professional advice are lost.

The elderly. The aim of treatment for the elderly is safe function in the activities of daily living. A few relevant exercises must be repeated in the same way each day during short treatment sessions. Balance and transfers are essential; stump exercises are of secondary importance. The elderly may tire more easily, have sensory or perceptual impairments, will undoubtedly have more than one disorder, and vascular amputees in particular may lose the remaining leg within 2 years and have a short life expectancy. The whole team must therefore work towards ensuring a quality of life in the remaining years which is acceptable to the patient.

IDEAS FOR THE EXERCISE PROGRAMME

Starting positions used

1. Sitting

The patient should be seated on a large plinth which is at the same height as the wheelchair to ensure safe transfer. Sitting balance must be achieved before anything else. The proprioceptive neuromuscular facilitation (PNF) technique of rhythmic stabilisation can be used, with manual contacts on the scapulae and pelvis. This can be progressed to throwing and catching exercises and a wobble board can be used (see Fig. 4.1).

Arm exercises should be carried out by all patients, particularly those with upper limb weakness. Exercises include push-up blocks (see Fig. 4.2) with which rhythmic stabilisations can again be performed. Weight and pulley systems can be used particularly effectively for graded bilateral resisted latissimus dorsi work. All patients must be able to push up in order to lift their buttocks off the bed or chair.

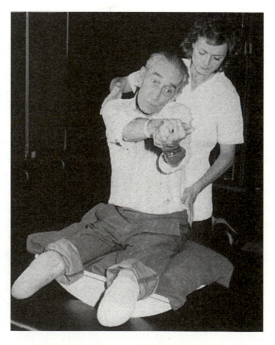

Fig. 4.1 Sitting wobble board exercise.

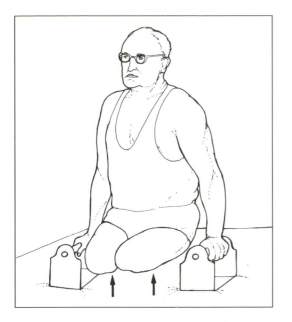

Fig. 4.2 A bilateral above-knee amputee using push-up blocks.

2. Supine lying

In this position the remaining leg, trunk and arms can be effectively treated in a variety of ways. PNF patterns to the remaining leg or upper limbs can be particularly useful to facilitate muscle work in order to increase strength and endurance. Also, using the principle of overflow, they can be used to facilitate muscle work on the amputated side. Once the most appropriate patterns have been selected, pulley and weight systems can be set up to provide the appropriate resistance so that the amputee can perform contractions (see Fig. 4.3).

The weight and number of contractions can be increased daily. This often gives the amputee, particularly the younger one, a measurable goal of achievement. Stump exercises can also be effectively performed in this position with manual assistance or resistance.

3. Side lying

Initially, many amputees require assistance to roll into this position. PNF patterns of the head, upper limb and trunk can be useful to facilitate the movement. With practice, many amputees will achieve this independently, although the very frail or those with other e.g. neurological, problems might not. This position is particularly useful for facilitating hip extension. Again PNF techniques of repeated contractions, plus hold, as

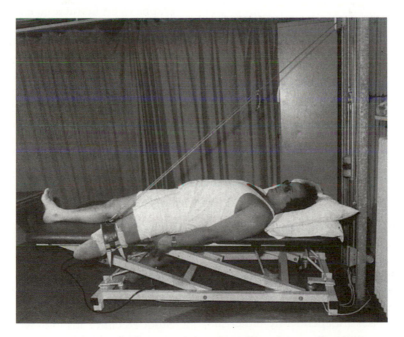

Fig. 4.3 Mechanically resisted exercise using a Westminster pulley system.

well as advanced repeated contractions can be useful, especially to re-educate the hip extensors and/or abductors. If hip extension is limited, hold–relax of the flexors can be performed in order to increase the range of extension.

4. Prone lying

It must be emphasised that patients with cardio-respiratory problems, kyphotic spines or gross arthritis will never be comfortable in this position; in which case it is inappropriate to choose this position for exercises.

For those patients who are able to tolerate lying prone it is a particularly effective position for arm exercises, e.g. press-ups, trunk and hip extension exercises.

5. Kneeling

Providing wound healing is complete, the below-knee and through-knee amputee, both unilateral and bilateral, can try to exercise in two-point or four-point kneeling or standing with the stump resting on a stool. The purpose is to improve balance reactions, weight transference and sensation in the stump to prepare for prosthetic use. It is hard exercise, and inappropriate for some elderly patients (Figs 4.4 and 4.5).

It is necessary in the early stages, particularly for the through-knee amputee, to place a soft covering over the stump, or to place a pillow under the stump to protect the skin while kneeling. Rhythmic stabilisations with progressive speed and resistance can be used.

Dynamic stump exercises

Dynamic stump exercises are simply multipurpose exercises combining the actions of the muscles of the stump with the rest of the body. They are used in the pre-prosthetic stage (and during any period when the prosthesis is not worn) to facilitate restoration of body symmetry. Some of these exercises are very hard and may not be suitable for the very elderly or frail. However, they can be adapted to suit most patients. Their advantage is that the patient can carry out these exercises independently either in the hospital ward or at home.

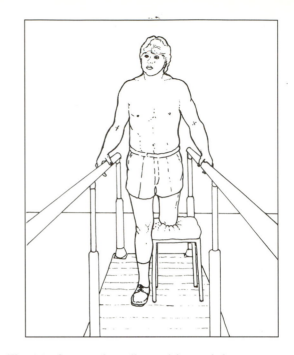

Fig. 4.4 Supported standing applying graded pressure to a through-knee stump.

Effects gained

1. The stump muscles are strengthened with emphasis on adductors, extensors and internal rotators.
2. The stump becomes accustomed to taking pressure, in preparation for prosthetic use.
3. The circulation is increased.
4. The flexibility of joints is maintained.
5. The muscle tone is promoted.
6. The patient's proprioceptive sense is re-educated in that the exercises at the same time involve movement of the rest of the body.
7. The patient learns the muscle coordination required of the stump in preparation for using a prosthesis.

Equipment

The following items are used:

1. Thick towels or pillows made into rolls of different sizes
2. Stool 18 cm (7 in) high with a soft padded top
3. Firm wide plinth

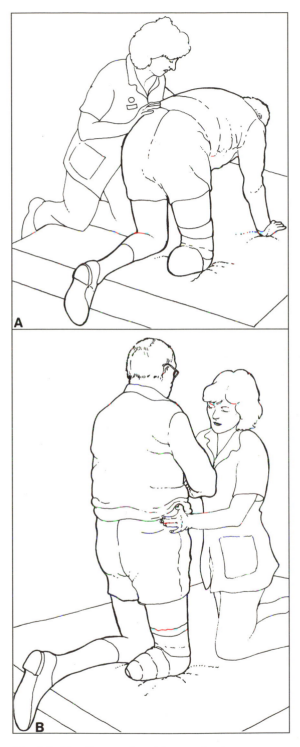

Fig. 4.5 Kneeling exercise with manual resistance.
(A) Four-point kneeling; (B) two-point kneeling.

Exercise 1. Stump extension with anterior pelvic thrust

Position (Fig. 4.6)

The patient lies supine with a pillow under the head. The stump is placed on a 18 cm (7 in) stool, with the opposite leg flexed (to reduce lumbar lordosis).

Movement

The patient presses the stump forcibly against the stool so that the hips are lifted off the mat and held there momentarily. The physiotherapist can either assist or resist the movement.

Purpose

The action is similar to that which occurs during the gait cycle as the prosthesis enters the support phase, and the remaining limb enters swing phase after the foot leaves the ground.

Exercise 2. Adduction of the internally rotated stump with lateral pelvic thrust

Position (Fig. 4.7)

The patient lies on the unaffected side with the stump resting on the stool; the opposite leg is flexed forwards and held up off the plinth. The

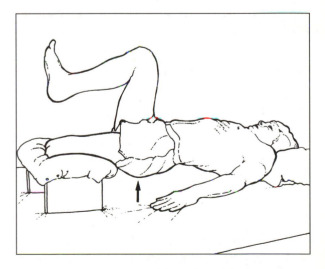

Fig. 4.6 Stump extension with anterior pelvic thrust.

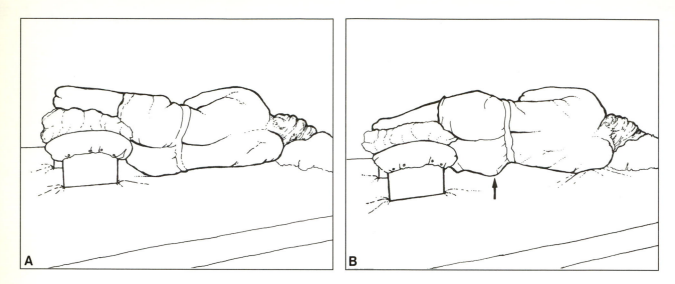

Fig. 4.7 Adduction of the internally rotated stump with lateral pelvic thrust.

trunk is stabilised by the arms. Some patients need an extra pillow on top of the stool.

Movement

The internally rotated stump is pushed strongly downwards into adduction, and the pelvis is elevated. The physiotherapist can either assist or resist the movement.

Some patients tend to roll forwards, thus elevating the rear rather than the side of the pelvis; the physiotherapist must then stabilise the upper shoulders and hips of the patient. Shoulder, hip and stump must then remain in a straight line.

Purpose

In the prosthetic gait cycle of the above-knee amputee there is a tendency to bend the trunk over the supporting side. The adductors and internal rotators should contract as weight is put on the prosthesis.

Exercise 3. Stump abduction with pelvic elevation

Position (Fig. 4.8)

The patient lies on the affected side. The stump is adducted with a stool, towelling roll or pillow placed under its abductor surface. The patient stabilises the position by using his arms.

Movement

The patient abducts the stump hard down on the stool or pillow until the pelvis is lifted. Extension must be maintained. Range can be increased by moving the stool or pillow distally.

Purpose

This exercise should prevent the Trendelenburg gait. Any patient who has not walked for a length of time will have weak hip abductors.

Exercise 4. Stump adduction with extension

Position (Fig. 4.9)

The patient lies prone, with the hips flat on the mat. A pillow or rolled towel is placed between the thighs.

Movement

The patient presses the thighs together and squeezes the roll. This causes simultaneous back and hip extension.

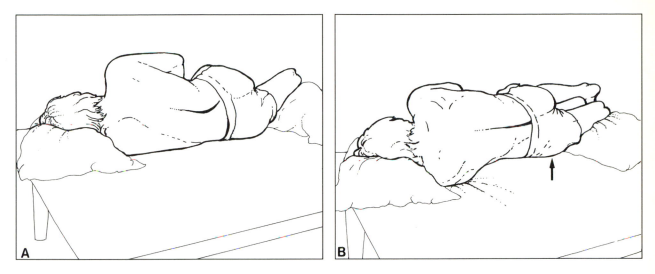

Fig. 4.8   Stump abduction with pelvic elevation.

Mechanically resisted exercises

Pulleys

A weight and pulley system can be used for arm or leg exercises, either to simulate the gait pattern or as an isolated movement. Any starting position can be used. Repetitive exercises can be carried out which help build up muscle endurance and general fitness. The weight and the number of repetitions can be increased daily. This often gives the younger amputee, in particular, a measurable goal of achievement.

Isokinetic exercise

In this type of exercise the speed of the muscular performance is controlled rather than the amount of resistance or the distance moved. Equipment used may be pre-set to hold the speed of a body movement at a constant rate, irrespective of the magnitude of forces generated by the participating muscles. The resistance offered by the machine matches the patient's immediate and specific muscular capacity of a body segment throughout a range of motion, but without per-

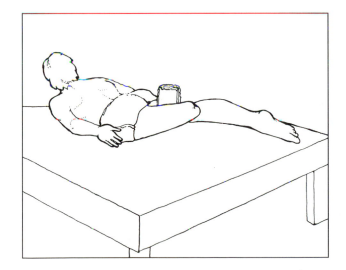

Fig. 4.9   Stump adduction with extension.

mitting acceleration to occur. This type of exercise is also termed accommodating resistance exercise.

The mounting of the isokinetic device is adjustable so that the lever arm can be positioned for movement in virtually any plane; a large variety of exercise patterns are thus possible.

The apparatus can be used in measurement of muscle performance with great accuracy and provide an objective measure of torque, total work and power rates for evaluation purposes. Examples of these systems are the Orthotron II and Cybex.

This type of exercise is particularly useful for the fitter amputee, who needs to exercise all four limbs. The lever arms may not accommodate knee or elbow flexion/extension with a short stump; however, they can be used for full hip and shoulder movements. Later in the patient's rehabilitation, when the stump is healed and prosthetic tolerance has been built up, the iso-kinetic systems can be used wearing the prosthesis (see Fig. 4.10).

Points to consider during the exercise programme

a. Patients can be treated both individually and in groups. A period of individual work daily will enable the physiotherapist to observe progress and to increase the exercise programme where appropriate. Communication between patient and therapist is on-going. Group work with other amputees or patients with different conditions is fun and of great psychological value.

Exercise classes can be given in a gymnasium area for the fitter patients. The physiotherapist must remain sensitive towards patients' feelings when they are being viewed in a group or class situation.

b. A programme of home exercises must be taught. It should include the most relevant exercises for each individual and must not be complicated. Generally, a maximum of five exercises is recommended. They should be written down in a form understandable to the patient.

c. The physiotherapist should always handle both the stump and remaining leg with care. The position of hand holds and mechanical resistance (of pulley harness, straps, sandbags, etc) must be considered. Damage to the tissues of the stump or remaining leg, particularly in the dysvascular patient, can easily occur if padding is inadequate.

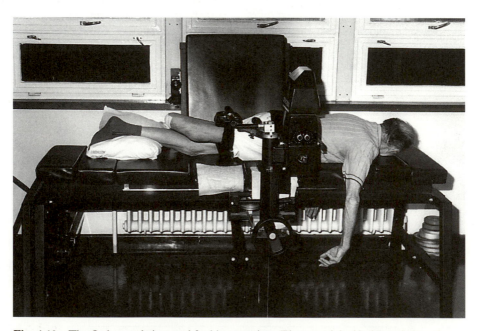

Fig. 4.10 The Orthotron being used for hip extension. (Photograph by kind permission of Mr H. Eldridge and VCMSM department of photography).

IDEAS FOR THE TREATMENT OF CONTRACTURES

Reasons for contractures

1. Contractures can occur pre-operatively as a result of pain and inactivity. The body's reaction to pain is to hold the limb in a flexed position. The contracture should be noted, measured and recorded pre-operatively by the physiotherapist. However, following amputation, the patient may maintain a flexed position through habit, muscle imbalance and immobility.

2. Specific joint problems (such as osteo-arthrosis and rheumatoid arthritis) may present with muscular, capsular and ligamentous tightness; the joint may be flared up in an acute phase. Furthermore, there may be permanent restriction of the joint caused by previous fractures or trauma.

3. If the patient is an established limb wearer and has to stop using the prosthesis for any reason for a period of time (see p. 37), contractures both at the hip and knee joints can develop through sitting for prolonged periods.

4. Pain which persists after the amputation will cause the limb to be held in flexion; analgesia should be reviewed and the cause investigated. If there is ischaemic pain, the amputation may not have been performed sufficiently proximally to ablate the disease, or the disease may have progressed. Also, with increasing age the established non-vascular amputee can develop peripheral vascular disease. The whole team must be aware of this problem: it is often the night nurse who observes the patient clasping the stump in flexion or dangling it over the edge of the bed to try to alleviate the pain (see Ch. 19).

Treatment

The techniques listed below are for both the prevention and treatment of contractures:

1. Active or resisted muscle work, either directly to the limb or to the rest of the body to gain overflow: proprioceptive neuromuscular facilitation techniques are particularly appropriate.

2. Diligent positioning of the stump or limbs to prevent contracture: the whole team must be aware of correct positions and constantly remind the patient. The prone or supine positions and use of stump boards, etc, are mentioned in Chapter 3.

3. Passive stretching: this must be performed with great care and sensitivity, particularly with regard to the underlying pathology. The physiotherapist should be experienced enough to 'feel' the end of the range, whether it is elastic or blocked.

To reduce existing contracture other modalities can be used depending on the pathology present:

a. Ice
b. Plaster-of-Paris or other rigid materials for serial splints
c. Passive mobilisations
d. Ultrasound therapy

Patients with contractures require frequent but short periods of treatment daily. Accurate measurement of the joint using a goniometer and noting the starting position used must be recorded at least weekly. It must be realised that treatment may only prevent the contracture getting worse, rather than improving it. These principles of treatment apply to contractures of joints in both the stump and the remaining limb, the difference being that there is inherent muscle imbalance in the stump.

IDEAS FOR THE TREATMENT OF ADHERENT SCARS

Adherent scars on the stump may result from slowly healing wounds or previous surgery to that limb. They can present problems with prosthetic fitting, especially when they immediately overlie a bony prominence. Treatment should commence when healing is complete and no open areas remain.

Treatment

1. Gentle thumb and finger massage, using a non-reactive cream, to mobilise the tissues.
2. Ultrasound, using a high frequency, low intensity beam directly over the scar. (The usual contra-indications to this treatment apply.)

CONTINUOUS ASSESSMENT

While the physiotherapist is treating the patient in the department, on-going assessment must take place. Observation of strength, movement, balance, perception, personality and interpersonal reactions will enable an accurate assessment of function to be made so that realistic goals of treatment can be planned.

It is most important that there is free communication between therapists and patients. The patient's wishes must be known and understood so that individual identity is preserved. Not all patients wish to achieve the goal the therapist has set for them. Weekly meetings with the other team members are important to communicate the patients' achievements and to plan their future progress. Ideally the whole team should assemble for case discussions but ward rounds can be attended for this purpose, or telephone calls made if attendance is impossible.

FUNCTIONAL ACTIVITY

Treatment for the lower limb amputee in the occupational therapy department is parallel to that in the physiotherapy department. The occupational therapist will have seen the patient in the early stages but will treat the patient on a daily basis when balance has improved. Occupational therapy provides activity and stimulation which are vital to the patients' recovery and will complement the skills learned in physiotherapy. Throughout the whole programme the therapist must see the patient within the context of the family and home situation.

Pre-prosthetic activities

1. Dressing practice

This is started in the ward immediately postoperatively but may be required on a continuous basis, especially for the elderly or confused patient. It is beneficial to show the carer how independent the patient can be so that this is maintained at home. It may be necessary to adapt clothing and special shoes.

2. Transfers

Functional transfers should be practised with:

— The bath with aids (Fig. 4.11)
— The toilet with clothing adjustment (Fig. 4.12)
— The bed
— The armchair.

3. Wheelchair activities

Some patients require daily practice in manoeuvring their wheelchair. If the patient is unlikely to

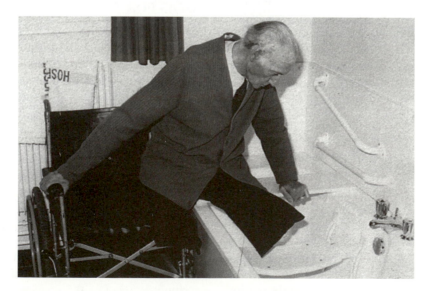

Fig. 4.11 Bath transfer. Note the position of the wheelchair with one arm rest removed. Bath board, inner bath seat and two grab rails are in situ.

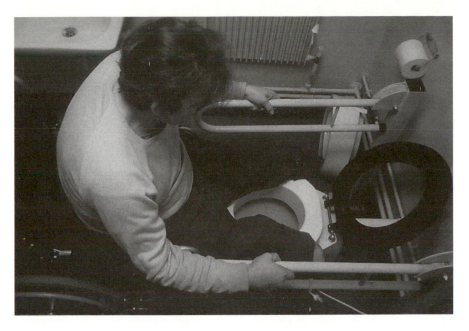

Fig. 4.12   A bilateral below-knee amputee doing a forward transfer onto the toilet.

be a prosthetic user, then a great deal more emphasis needs to be put on this activity to ensure that domestic independence can be achieved from a wheelchair. Outdoor mobility should be practised on different surfaces for those patients with sufficient exercise tolerance.

4. Arm strengthening exercises

Some activities are directed towards upper limb strengthening while others enable the patient to gain skills and confidence in independent living. Included here are printing, gardening, woodwork, washing and ironing personal clothing, and cooking (see Fig. 4.13). These activities need to be individually graded to each patient's needs.

5. Self-expression

It is often when the patient is engaged in a familiar activity that personal feelings may begin to be expressed, either to the therapist or to another patient. The less rushed and less clinical atmosphere lends itself to quiet discussion which should be seen as an adjunct to specialist counselling help.

6. Home visits

There are different purposes for the home visit,

depending on the stage in the rehabilitation process. Visits provide an excellent opportunity to discuss mobility, independence and other issues with relatives.

1. Early home assessment

This can take place either pre-operatively or very early postoperatively. The rehabilitation staff visit the home to gain information about the environment in order to:

— Order an appropriate wheelchair if necessary
— Ascertain the need for any aids and
    adaptations
— Formulate a realistic rehabilitation plan.

2. Home visit

This is done with hospital staff and the patient in order to see whether sufficient functional independence has been achieved. Local social service and district nursing personnel may wish to be present as well, as communication with the local authority agencies is vital.

   At this stage the patient may be mobile in the wheelchair, hopping with crutches or frame, mobile with the prosthesis or any combination of these. All transfers, wheelchair manoeuvrability,

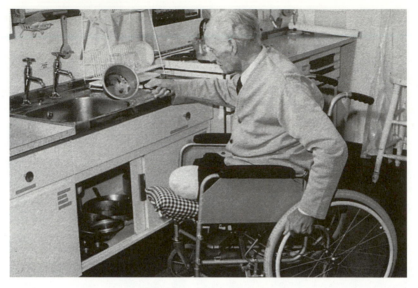

Fig. 4.13   Cooking practice.

donning and doffing the prosthesis, step and stair climbing need to be carried out during the visit (see Fig. 4.14).

3. Follow-up visit

This visit is carried out soon after discharge, either from hospital or from an out-patient programme, to ensure that the maximum independence gained is being maintained with safety.

Hospital, DSC or community therapists, outreach teams or social services may visit, depending on local availability of services and factors identified as continuing needs before discharge.

Prosthetic activities

When the patient is confident in standing and is beginning to walk outside the parallel bars, functional walking can be commenced and more complicated standing activities. Work in the kitchen is applicable to most patients and practice of a familiar and necessary activity will build confidence. If the patient uses walking aids, the use of a trolley in order to move food and drink from one room to another will need to be explored (Fig. 4.15). Standing practice is of particular importance to bilateral amputees (see Ch. 16).

More active patients benefit from more vigorous activities such as woodwork (see Fig. 4.16) or

gardening, involving transferring weight evenly, reaching up and down, sitting on the floor,

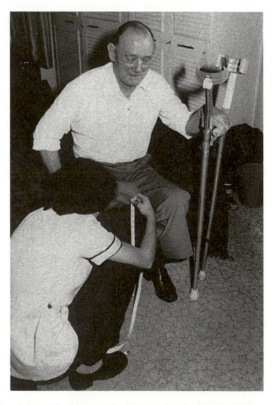

Fig. 4.14   The home visit. All functional activities in the home are checked both with and without the prosthesis.

kneeling and getting up, and lifting objects. Walking outside in public environments, e.g. pavements, crossing roads, entering shops and buildings, using public transport, stairs and escalators (Fig. 4.17), should be practised with a therapist first, so that possible hazards are identified and overcome before the patient attempts them alone. A familiar and regular journey such as going to school or work is the most relevant activity to undertake, even though this may take time and effort on behalf of the therapist or their community based colleague because double or triple the previous journey time needs to be allowed.

SOCIAL WORK

In assessing the patient in social and psychological terms it must always be remembered that no two patients are going to react in the same way. There are general attitudes and stages which patients encounter during their acceptance of the physical changes they undergo, but the timing of each phase varies with each patient and can never be fully anticipated.

If the social worker is to understand the patient's progress in physical and psychological terms then the patient's performance should be observed at appropriate intervals. Reinforcement of positive progress can be shared if the social worker visits the physiotherapy and occupational therapy departments. More importantly, if the patient is presenting with a negative attitude towards treatment after amputation, this will have to be explored.

Obviously, there are many patients who cope with amputation within their own limits and only require guidance and support, and this not necessarily from the social workers. However, there are others who feel quite shocked following amputation and require specialised help. These patients often withdraw, feeling that their whole social world has been altered to such a degree that to continue the struggle would be too overwhelming. Their dependence and hopelessness can

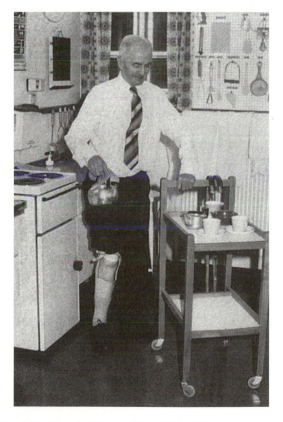

Fig. 4.15 Practice of an activity of daily living using a patellar tendon bearing (PTB) temporary prosthesis.

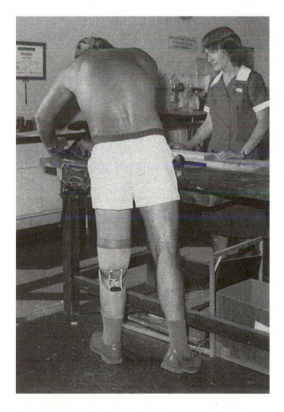

Fig. 4.16 Woodwork activity in the occupational therapy heavy workshop.

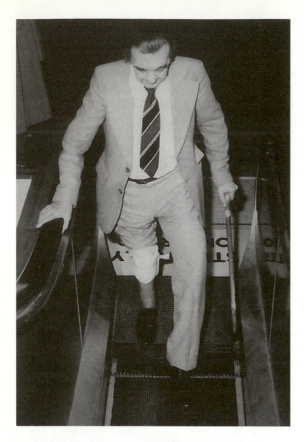

Fig. 4.17   A below-knee amputee using an escalator.

present in overt depression, anger, and more commonly regression. The impact of amputation may drastically alter the balance of interpersonal relationships, and cause loss of status within a family unit. Regular counselling with the patient and family prevent considerable misunderstanding of assumed expectations and lead to a clearer and more honest knowledge of how the patient is feeling and coping with the amputation and changes in lifestyle. The anxieties related to how they are going to re-establish themselves and regain confidence can sometimes become overwhelming and the result can be immobilising. Regular counselling can never totally prevent this reaction, but it can allow the patient to deal with it in stages, recognising the fact that some responsibility can be taken for their own social future.

Amputation is unlikely to create totally new psychological states in the patient; it may, however, heighten some of the more neurotic, obsessional, histrionic or depressive qualities which were present in the patient's psychological make-up prior to amputation. Some of these symptoms will decrease as independence is attained and achievements accomplished; others may require medication to decrease the immobilising effects of the patient's psychological condition. In the more severe cases of denial and depression, psychiatric opinion should be sought. The psychological defences are often used unconsciously, giving the patient time to come to terms with the destructive surgery and disturbing experience. Whilst the patient is receiving physiotherapy and occupational therapy, counselling should continue at the same pace, thus reinforcing the patient's attainments, however minor.

REFERENCES

Alpert S H 1982 The psychological aspects of amputation surgery. Orthotics and Prosthetics 36(4): 50–56

Baruch I M, Mossberg K A 1983 Heart-rate response of elderly women to nonweight-bearing ambulation with a walker. Physical Therapy 63(11): 1782–1787

Chadwick S J D 1986 Restoring dignity and mobility in the amputee. Geriatric Medicine 16(7): 43–46

Eisert O, Tester O W 1954 Dynamic exercises for lower extremity amputees. Archives of Physical Medicine and Rehabilitation 35: 695–704

Furst L, Humphrey M 1983 Coping with the loss of a leg. Prosthetics and Orthotics International 7: 152–156

Kavanagh T, Shephard R J 1973 The application of exercise testing to the elderly amputee. Canadian Medical Association Journal 108: 314–317

Moncur S D 1969 The practical aspect of balance relating to amputees. Physiotherapy 55(2): 409–410

Moverley L 1990 Discovering water's redeeming features. Therapy Weekly 17(7): 4

Parkes C M 1972 Components of the reaction to loss of a limb, spouse or home. Journal of Psychosomatic Research 16: 343–349

Thompson D M, Haran D 1984 Living with an amputation: the patient. International Rehabilitation Medicine 5(4): 165–169

Tilbury B 1981 Some general thoughts on the rehabilitation of the elderly amputee. Newsletter of the Demonstration Centres in Rehabilitation 26: 44–52

5. Early mobility

Achieving an independent means of moving around early in the rehabilitation programme, either in a wheelchair, hopping or walking with simple aids, has many obvious advantages for both elderly and young amputees: no longer having to rely on others for basic daily needs (such as going to the toilet) is of great psychological benefit. To be able to stand up to converse with others and to feel able to walk again, even if it is only for short distances, gives the amputee a great sense of achievement. The patient is also reassured that greater mobility will soon be possible.

Patients carry out regular progressive exercise programmes both in the physiotherapy and occupational therapy departments. Independent wheelchair activities and the use of the Ppam aid commence within the first 2 weeks postoperatively. Hopping is not encouraged until the stump is healed.

WHEELCHAIR MOBILITY

Wheelchair loan

A wheelchair is loaned to the amputee in the early postoperative period as a means of mobility. This is because it is essential not to cause dependent oedema of the stump at this stage, and balance with standing and hopping can be difficult for the elderly. The remaining foot may also have fragile tissue viability and be unable to take vertical and shear forces.

The benefits of using a wheelchair at this stage include upper limb strengthening, increased cardiorespiratory output, increased stamina and independence in the activities of daily living. Early mobility also gives a psychological boost to the amputee.

The physiotherapist must also be aware of the identification that exists in people's minds linking the wheelchair with disability: patients may suffer a depressive reaction from using this symbol of disability in the early postoperative phase and this needs to be addressed in a positive manner by the multidisciplinary team.

For some patients, the wheelchair may be the only method of mobility: bilateral amputees rely heavily on their wheelchairs and some unilateral amputees who are frail or weak, have cardio-respiratory, neurological or arthritic disease, and are unable to hop with safety, may also rely solely on their wheelchairs. However, the choice of using the wheelchair should remain with the patient once the advantages and disadvantages have been explained.

Wheelchair assessment

The amputee will have been loaned a suitable and safe self-propelling wheelchair immediately postoperatively. Once the patient's medical condition has stabilised and an early home assessment (see Ch. 4) has been carried out, the need for, and prescription of, a permanent wheelchair should be addressed. Many standard works have been written about the prescription of wheelchairs and seating to which the therapist should refer (see Bibliography), along with information from the district wheelchair service, suppliers and approved repairer.

Assessment criteria

The following is an outline only of assessment considerations as they relate to the amputee (see Fig. 5.1).

1. *Patient*

— Body proportions
— Skin condition, particularly of pressure areas
— Cognitive and perceptual function
— Manual dexterity and coordination
— Posture and presence of any deformity, particularly of spine and hips; any asymmetry, particularly hip disarticulation and hemipelvectomy
— Ability to lift up, transfer and balance
— Site of amputation; uni- or bilateral; prognosis and likelihood of any further surgery in the future
— Weight distribution in the chair and liability to tip over backwards
— Prosthetic design and suspension, if used
— Patient's preferences and lifestyle.

WHEEL&HAIRS
Wheelchair Education and Training Group

CHECKLIST
Assessment, Prescription, Provision and Review

1. Establish the reason for referral and the client's/parents'/carers' wishes.

2. Observe the current prescription of wheelchair/seating and the way that the client is using these.

3. Assess, measure and/or record the client's posture and function in current equipment.

4. With client out of equipment examine the components and their condition.

5. Assess the client in positions of lying, sitting and standing in order to determine his abilities in each of these positions. **Do not use prescribed equipment for this process**.

6. Measure and note presence of deformity, particularly of the spine and hips, taking care to check for any asymmetric deformities. Determine whether deformity is fixed or postural and the degree of correction achievable.

7. Define pressure distribution needs.

8. Determine the treatment/management programmes related to the client's postural support needs.

9. Determine environmental and social constraints on the prescriptions.

10. Use the collected data to determine the posture (upright or alternatives) and the support required by the client. Simulate this support with the aim of drafting the prescription, bearing in mind the following:

10a. **For tissue trauma considerations**, determine the appropriate pressure distributing or pressure re-distributing cushion either commercially available or purpose made.

10b. **For postural considerations**, whenever possible,
  i. Aim for symmetry and distribution of load bearing through both ischial tuberosities and the whole of the thighs and buttocks.
  ii. Avoid pelvic tilt, ie. pelvis to be neutral.
  iii. Avoid asymmetry, eg. windswept hips, scoliosis, etc.
  iv. Provide appropriate support to stabilize the pelvis and lower limbs in all the postures being considered.
  v. Once the lower part of the body has been stabilized, determine the postural support required at the trunk level without diminishing functional ability.

11. Use support surfaces that provide bio-mechanically correct application of forces (references 1, 2, 3, 6).

12. If the foregoing is not readily achievable, referral to a specialist centre is required.

13. Choose, or design and manufacture (an iterative process), the most appropriate support system to provide the bio-mechanically correct postural stability to achieve the above objectives. The equipment should preferably be adjustable to meet the changing needs of the client.

14. Determine the type of wheeled mobility into which this postural support system will fit and which will also be compatible with the client's lifestyle, the family's/carer's lifestyles, physical abilities and mental abilities. Consider the following:
  a, Self propelled, attendant propelled or powered mobility.
  b, Indoor or outdoor or both.
  c, Size - open and folded (for seating system, access to buildings, transportation, space, convenience).
  d, Need for various components to be removable.
  e, Weight with or without removable components.
  f, Ease of use including manoeuvrability and removable components.
  g, Footrest position with reference to sitting posture.
  h, Castor position with reference to desired foot position.
  i, Stability of chair with occupant.
  j, The wheelchair or other wheeled mobility devices should permit the full range of adjustment of the postural support equipment.

15. Determine whether or not provision is through NHS or by private purchase using published lists of wheelchairs and other vehicles.

16. The prescribed wheelchair must be tested for static stability with client in place. If unstable, determine modifications required or new prescription and retest on completion.

17. Instruct the client and/or carers in the particular features and functions of the seating system and wheelchair(s) and other vehicle(s), including maintenance and responsibilities for correct use.

18. Identify intervals for review and set dates.

Roy Nelham, Carolyn Nichols, Pauline Pope   1989

Fig. 5.1 Wheelchair checklist. Reproduced courtesy of Roy Nelham, Carolyn Nichols and Pauline Pope (1989).

2. *Environment*

— Home and work: to include access and egress, turning space, work and storage unit heights, storage space for chair
— Leisure and social requirements, including transport
— Carer's ability, availability, preferences and lifestyle.

3. *Use*

— Occasional: e.g. when fatigued, when not wearing the prosthesis, or when the tissue viability of the remaining limb is compromised
— Permanent: e.g. bilateral amputees or when prosthetic rehabilitation is not possible or wanted

— Could the mobility need be met in other ways? e.g. taxi card and Dial-a-Ride.

4. *Maintenance*

— Tyre inflation pressure
— Routine oiling and ease of moving any removable parts
— Function of brakes
— State of repair of canvas
— State of cushion/seating
— Maintenance and recharging of battery (powered chairs)
— Is the patient or the carer able to perform these tasks and has he or she been trained? Does the patient or carer have the relevant telephone numbers of the local wheelchair provision centre and the approved repairer?

Hardware

This is obtained from the local wheelchair clinic, where a variety of models of chair can be tried out and where specialist therapists and technical staff can provide expert assessment and advice.

1. *Chair*

— Self-propelling lightweight folding chairs are usually prescribed for amputees (see Fig. 5.2)
— Powered chairs may be prescribed if exercise tolerance is low and/or the chair is for permanent use
— Accessories
  • Removable arm rests
  • Safety belts
  • Swinging detachable foot rests
  • Stump board (see Ch. 3)
  • Rear wheels set back 3 ins for unilateral amputees who are unstable, i.e. likely to tip backwards on an incline, and for all bilateral amputees. This will increase the wheelbase and thus, a larger turning circle is required. This is important to consider in small areas such as lifts in blocks of flats, offices, etc.

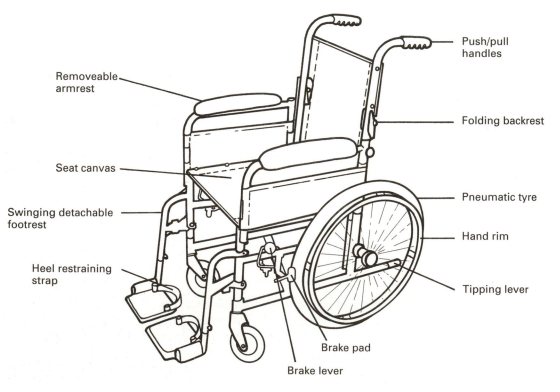

Fig. 5.2 A self-propelling wheelchair

2. *Cushion*
— Standard 2 in, 3 in or 4 in foam
— Sheepskin
— Plywood base
— Check that the cushion remains in place on transfers, particularly with bilateral amputees
— Special cushions are available if standard ones have been tried and do not meet the needs of the amputee, e.g. a heavy gel cushion is sometimes suitable for bilateral amputees as it will not wrinkle during a sliding or shuffling transfer and will provide suitable pressure area protection.

3. *Other*

— Private supply: financial support is available from a variety of statutory or charitable organisations; details should be obtained from the local wheelchair clinic. Some patients prefer to purchase their own chairs.
— Lightweight high performance chairs for young, high level bilateral amputees are popular.
— Outdoor powered chairs: very careful and specialist assessment is required before purchase. This may be obtained from the Mobility Advice and Vehicle Information Service, Department of Transport, Disabled Living Foundation, Keep Able, etc. (see Appendix for addresses.)

Instruction to patient and carer

Independent wheelchair activities will be part of the rehabilitation programme in the physiotherapy and occupational therapy departments (see Chs 3 and 4). Suitable parking positions for toilet and bed transfers are identified and the patient practises manipulating the wheelchair through doorways, into lifts, around corners, on carpets and ramps. Further practice takes place on the home visit.

Education is given in safety checking and routine maintenance, and information written down and given concerning when and from where further advice should be obtained.

Both the amputee and the carer should be shown how to fold and unfold the chair correctly and how to lift the chair, paying due attention to back care. Negotiation of steps and kerbs must be practised to find the safest and least strenuous method that both feel comfortable using.

Reassessment

Patients who have been supplied with a wheelchair may need review appointments. Individual needs alter over time, particularly for those with chronic progressive disease such as peripheral vascular disease and diabetes. For the amputee, the general decline of strength and mobility with increasing age and possible accommodation change, can be compounded by weight change, more proximal amputation of the existing stump, loss of the remaining limb and a decline in cardiopulmonary function with consequent loss of exercise tolerance. Reassessment of the prescription and/or adaptations thus needs to be made and re-ordering of a permanent chair, return to a loan scheme or private purchase should be considered. The community physiotherapist is frequently the team member best placed to monitor changes and initiate the process whereby prescription review can be carried out.

HOPPING

Hopping is initially taught in the parallel bars. The younger patient will then progress to using crutches with ease. The more elderly patient will probably manage to stand up on the remaining leg; some may hop using the bars or a walking frame if there is adequate upper limb strength together with reasonable balance and coordination.

The purpose of achieving hopping with an aid is that the patient will have an alternative method of mobility about the home. Going to the toilet and bathroom early in the morning and late in the evening is often easier without the prosthesis. Access to these areas in the wheelchair is not always possible so the ability to hop short distances is frequently essential. If there is a mechanical breakdown of the prosthesis or tissue damage of the stump, the patient must either hop or use the wheelchair.

Too much hopping at an early stage in the rehabilitation programme may be inadvisable because:

a. The stump is dependent; therefore oedema, discomfort and pain may result.

b. The vascular patient may have an ischaemic and fragile remaining foot through which the sudden force of full weightbearing during hopping is dangerous and inadvisable.

c. Prolonged hopping, especially with the younger patient, may cause temporary postural defects such as pelvic tilt and spinal rotation. It can also be dangerous when hopping at high speeds as the stump can be carelessly knocked.

d. Many of the elderly patients are unwilling to stand and hop, not only because of physical problems, but because they feel unsafe and lack confidence.

e. A new bilateral amputee must not try to hop using the original prosthesis. It is unsafe and puts too great a stress through the soft tissues of the stump. Standing transfers, using the prosthesis, may be possible for a previous below-knee amputee.

An alternative to hopping is toe/heel swivelling. This has the advantages of requiring less arm strength and giving greater stability as the foot is always in contact with the floor. The danger for the dysvascular patient is large shear forces on the plantar soft tissues.

Patients will often find their own solutions to mobility needs, and those who feel unsafe hopping, or who cannot gain access using a wheelchair, may shuffle around on their bottom. Stairs may be accessible this way rather than by any other means.

THE PNEUMATIC POST AMPUTATION MOBILITY AID (Ppam Aid)

This partial weightbearing early walking aid must only be used under clinical supervision in the physiotherapy treatment area. It is not for ward or home use.

The aid can be used from 5–7 days post-operatively while the sutures are still in the wound, provided the surgeon is satisfied that wound healing is progressing satisfactorily and has given permission for its use, and the physiotherapist has observed the state of the wound.

It consists of a basic frame (in three lengths), two inflatable air bags which surround the stump,

and a foot pump (Fig. 5.3). The Pneumatic Post Amputation Mobility Aid is manufactured in Great Britain by Vessa Limited who produce a leaflet, free on request, describing the equipment and method of application for the below-knee amputee.

Advantages and disadvantages

The advantages of the Ppam aid are:

a. The great psychological boost gained by walking very soon after amputation.

b. The ability to assess the patient in terms of prosthetic fitting and rehabilitation prospects. Particular examples of this are the hemiplegic patient and those with severe cardiorespiratory disease. Mild confusional states often improve once standing and walking commence.

c. The reduction of oedema. As weight is taken through the amputated side the pressure in the bags is increased, and when weight is removed the pressure decreases. This pumping action

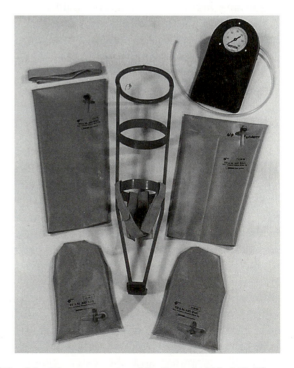

Fig. 5.3 The components of the Ppam Aid Mark II. The below-knee and through-knee bags are on the left of the metal frame; the above-knee bag is on the right.

reduces oedema and promotes wound healing. The support that the inflated plastic bags offer provides comfort for the dependent stump.

d. By encouraging partial weightbearing at an early stage, postural reactions are re-educated. This is important for those who have not stood up or walked for a long period of time prior to amputation. Muscle control of the trunk, remaining limb and hip on the amputated side are stimulated and balance is improved.

e. Preparation of the stump for the harder socket of a prosthesis is achieved by maintaining pressure around the stump. This also may help in reducing phantom sensation.

The disadvantages of the Ppam aid are:

a If a fixed knee flexion contracture is present, the stump is more liable to break down. The anterior aspect of the knee may rub against the metal frame, and there can be excessive pressures on the distal end of the stump.

b. Where there are fractures present in the femur (whether internally fixed or not) sufficient union or stability must be present to permit partial weightbearing. However, it must be remembered that rotational stress may occur while using the somewhat unstable Ppam aid. It may be safer to wait until the prosthesis can be supplied. If there is any doubt, the orthopaedic surgeon must be contacted.

c. If the patient is very heavy, or has a 'heavy footed' gait, excessive pistoning may occur and there will be insufficient support.

d. The experienced limb wearer who has further surgery to the stump finds partial weightbearing difficult, and may try to use the Ppam aid as a normal prosthesis.

Method of application of the Ppam aid for the below-knee and through-knee levels

a. The patient is fully dressed and sits on a firm chair inside the parallel bars. The stump dressing or bandage remains in place.

b. The physiotherapist inflates the small bag, no more than one-quarter full, invaginates it and places it over the distal end of the stump and trousers, if worn. The patient is asked to hold this in place. If the patient has a large stump, or

bulky dressings are present, the small bag is folded in half, slightly inflated, and held against the distal end of the stump.

c. The large bag (uninflated) is pulled over the stump and small bag, ensuring a smooth fit right up to the groin and buttock crease.

d. The correct size frame is eased up over the two bags and stump until it is about 8 cm from the top of the large bag.

e. The webbing straps are then fixed so that support is given to the distal end of the large bag.

f. The patient is asked to straighten the knee of the remaining leg so that a check of the length of the frame can be made.

g. The large bag is then inflated using the foot pump to approximately 40 mmHg pressure.

h. The patient then stands in the parallel bars and the fit of the Ppam aid is checked before balance exercise and walking are started.

Method of application of the Ppam aid for the above-knee stump (Fig. 5.4)

a. The patient starts in the same position as for the previous method.

b. The large bag for the above knee stump is pulled over the stump with the inflation tube on the lateral side.

c. The small bag (the same as for the below-knee and through-knee stumps) is folded in half and is slightly inflated. This is then pushed up inside the larger bag so that it touches the distal end of the stump (see Fig. 5.4A).

d. The frame is eased up over the large bag and the patient holds it in place; the length is checked with the remaining leg (see Fig. 5.4B).

e. The large bag is semi-inflated just enough so that it is held in position by the frame.

f. The patient then stands up on the remaining leg but is instructed NOT to bear weight yet through the Ppam aid. At this stage the physiotherapist pulls the large bag up as high as possible anteriorly and posteriorly (see Fig. 5.4C) and adjusts the length of the frame. The webbing straps may or may not be in a position to support the bags, depending on the length of the stump.

g. The outer bag is then inflated to 40 mmHg pressure using the foot pump.

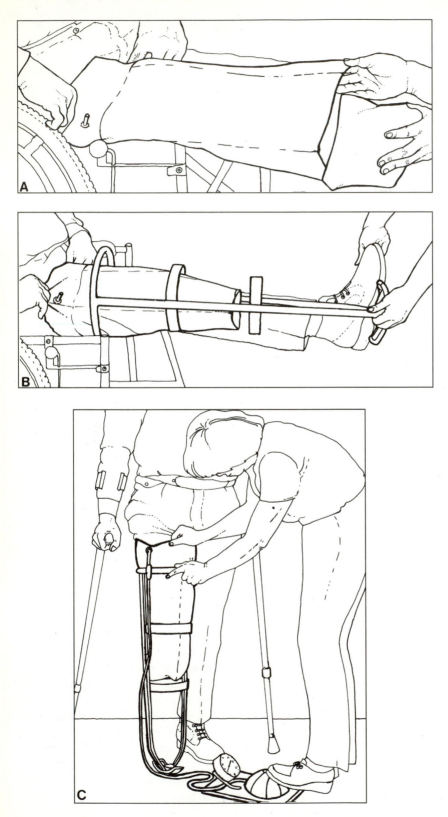

Fig. 5.4   Method of application of the Ppam aid for the above-knee stump.

h. The shoulder strap gives added suspension, passing over the opposite shoulder to the amputated side.

NB. The position of the above-knee Ppam aid may need frequent adjustment during the treatment session.

Use of the Ppam aid

a. It is recommended for patients whose wounds still have sutures in, show slow healing, or for those with low Doppler readings, that the Ppam aid is used only to stand up in briefly and possibly walk once the length of the parallel bars for the initial treatment sessions. For patients whose wounds are healed but are still tender, it is recommended that for the first 2–3 days the Ppam aid is not worn for more than 1 hour with frequent rest periods, during which time the bags are deflated and the patient's stump is elevated. For patients whose stumps have healed satisfactorily with no signs of ischaemia, this treatment time can be increased up to 2 hours with less frequent rest periods. While the patient is sitting down resting between walking or standing periods, the large bag must be deflated to reduce constant pressure on the new wound and the Ppam aid should be elevated.

b. The condition of the wound must be checked under sterile conditions daily, before and after treatment. Some oozing may have occurred or the dressing may have slipped and wound toilet or a new dressing will be required.

c. The elderly should always remain in the parallel bars. The younger patient with full strength in the upper limbs and good balance may progress from the parallel bars to walking with crutches. However, stair climbing, steps and slopes must not be attempted as the Ppam aid is only a partial weightbearing device. The Ppam aid should never be used with walking sticks.

d. It is possible for bilateral amputees who have previously been successful single amputees to use the Ppam aid, providing they are strong and can balance, with their existing prosthesis. It may be necessary to reduce the length of the original prosthesis to lower the centre of gravity in order to assist balance and mobility.

At Roehampton two Ppam aids are never used on bilateral amputees because excessive pistoning occurs within the plastic bags and tissue breakdown can follow. There is insufficient stability for the patient in two Ppam aids.

TRAINING AND TEMPORARY PROSTHESES

Above knee: the Femurett (Fig. 5.5)

The LIC Femurett provides greater stability than the Ppamaid for the above-knee amputee. There is an ischial seating area, firm lateral wall, basic knee mechanism and foot. The socket comes in different sizes and can be easily adjusted to the patient. There is a basic alignment device. The wound must be sufficiently healed to commence walking with a rigid socket.

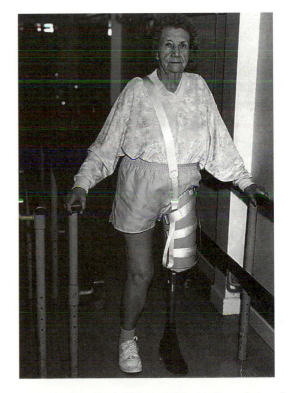

Fig. 5.5 The Femurett. (Photograph by kind permission of Mrs M. Boultwood., LIC and Dr Morrison, Oxford DSC.)

Below-knee: the Tulip Limb (Fig. 5.6)

The LIC Tulip Limb is a training device which can be used when the wound is sufficiently healed to tolerate a firm interface. It consists of an inner inflatable sac and an outer rigid shell socket, with shank and foot attached. As with the Ppam aids, the patient walks with a rigid knee.

The AK/BK temporary prosthesis (Fig. 5.7)

This temporary prosthesis is custom made by a prosthetist and is ischial weightbearing. A knee lock is present and the patient walks with a stiff knee gait. It is only supplied for the following reasons:

— An unhealed stump, e.g. burns, skin grafts, open wounds, infection, dermatological conditions
— An unstable knee joint
— An excessively hypersensitive or painful stump

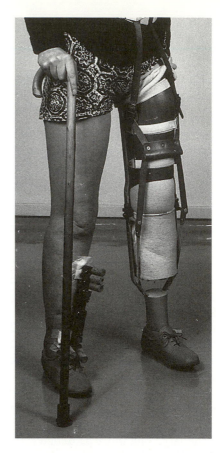

Fig. 5.7   The above-knee/below-knee temporary prosthesis. This patient has a skin graft on the distal end of the below-knee stump and a compound fracture of the contralateral tibia and fibula. Note the external fixator in situ.

— Fractures in the femur or tibial stump in the process of healing
— Knee flexion contracture more than 25°.

The advantage of this temporary prosthesis is that the patient can be measured for it pre-operatively and therefore postoperative mobility is hastened. This prevents the complications resulting from a sedentary or bedfast existence, and enables early discharge from hospital, even though healing is still in progress. The disadvantages are that it is cosmetically very unacceptable and difficult to apply. The quadriceps muscle is inhibited and the knee joint is immobilised. Furthermore, it may restrict the blood supply to a potentially ischaemic stump.

The construction of this temporary prosthesis is given below.

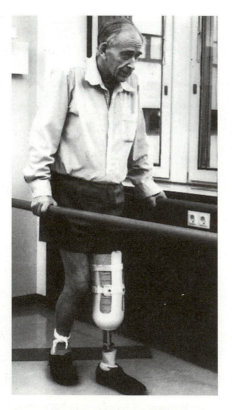

Fig. 5.6   The Tulip Limb.

Thigh corset

There is a blocked leather, front-fastening thigh corset which partially supports the body weight; the principal weight transmission area is the ischial seating area on the posterior aspect of the corset.

Suspension

The two types of suspension used are either a rigid pelvic band with shoulder strap or soft suspension (see Ch. 11).

Knee

This is a uniaxial joint with a simple spring device which locks the prosthesis in extension. A manual release, either H-strap or metal bar design, enables the amputee to sit with a flexed knee.

Socket

This is made of soft felt with a pad for distal tissue support. It is made sufficiently large to allow the stump to be properly bandaged in order to prevent dependent oedema. The felt socket protects the stump as the patient walks. No weight is transmitted through this felt socket, which should be regarded merely as a 'stump container'.

Base

This can be either a uniaxial or SACH foot (see Ch. 7).

Check of the above-knee/below-knee temporary prosthesis

The fit of the temporary prosthesis must be checked by the physiotherapist on the first attendance for gait re-education and subsequently at regular intervals. The patient's skin must be checked before and after each session.

Corset

With the patient standing and suitably undressed the physiotherapist should check the ischial seating and the adductor region in the following ways.

The ischial seating is checked for correct weightbearing as described in Chapter 11. The leather corset is checked for correct fastening.

If the ischium is not seated correctly the reason may be that:

a. The corset is too large: this is determined if the sides of the front opening are touching. To remedy this, more stump socks can be added of a variety of thicknesses.

b. The corset is too small: this is determined if the tongue of the leather is not covering the front opening. To remedy this, the number of stump socks and or their thickness can be reduced. It must be noted that the thigh corset must never be tighter proximally than distally as this constricts circulation.

If adjustments are still needed, the physiotherapist should contact the prosthetist.

Adductor region. There should be no discomfort in this area. Possible causes of discomfort may be that:

a. The patient is 'sinking' into the corset, which is probably a result of incorrect weightbearing on the ischium, or incorrect fastening of the leather corset.

b. The stump sock is inadequately pulled up over the rim of the corset.

c. There is insufficient strength and function of the hip extensor muscles on the affected side, causing the patient to flex at the hip and rub the skin area over the adductor region.

This can be a particularly common complaint by patients wearing such a temporary prosthesis. If further adjustments are necessary the physiotherapist should contact the prosthetist. The physiotherapist should not be tempted to pad or cut down the adductor region of the socket, as this does not reduce the discomfort.

Length

Standing. The prosthesis may be about 2 cm shorter than the natural leg to allow hitch-through during the swing phase. The method of checking the length is similar to that used for the above-knee prosthesis (see Ch. 11).

A common fault occurs when the patient has fastened the stump either 'in' or 'out' of the corset, thus making the prosthesis either too long or too short.

Sitting. The patient's knee should be free to flex to 90°. If the corset of the felt socket interferes with this action, the position of the stump within the socket should again be checked. The hinges of the prosthetic knee joint should lie about 1.5 cm above the knee joint line. (This is because the centre of rotation of the knee is situated near the centre of the medial femoral condyle.) If the prosthesis is incorrectly positioned, the anterior aspect of the stump will knock against the felt socket when the patient is seated.

Felt socket

This should not constrict the stump: it is important to remember that the below-knee stump must be bandaged in this temporary prosthesis. There should be tissue support distally in the container. The restraining straps around the container prevent excessive flexion during walking.

If the patient complains of discomfort in this area the physiotherapist should check that:

a. The socket is not too tight. Tightness may be a result of an oedematous stump or an excessive amount of dressing or bandage, which may be reduced.

b. The stump sock has not wrinkled within the socket and is causing constriction of the stump.

c. The prosthesis has been properly applied with the patient's knee extended fully so that the stump becomes correctly positioned within the socket.

If adjustments are still needed then the physiotherapist should contact the prosthetist.

Suspension

The method of checking the rigid pelvic band and shoulder strap is similar to that used for the above-knee prosthesis (see Ch. 11).

The soft suspension must be comfortable and the down straps from the belt to the socket must be firm when the patient is standing up. Very occasionally this temporary prosthesis is self-suspending, in which case the physiotherapist should check that there is no excessive pistoning between the patient's leg and the prosthesis during walking. This is best observed posteriorly with the patient walking away from the physiotherapist. If this occurs, the fastening on the corset should be checked to ensure that it is firm. On no account should the physiotherapist or patient tighten the corset so much that the stump becomes 'strangled', producing a tourniquet effect. This will damage the stump and prevent healing. If pistoning continues, auxiliary suspension is required and an appointment at the prosthetist must be made.

Knee lock

Before the patient applies the prosthesis, the physiotherapist should check the working of the knee lock mechanism to ensure that it locks and releases efficiently. The patient should be observed operating the lock to ensure that the process is fully understood. With the elderly this may take several sessions to achieve.

Functional re-education with the above-knee/below-knee temporary prosthesis

Application

1. The patient should sit on a firm bed, undressed apart from a vest.
2. The below-knee stump bandage must be in place (Fig. 5.8A).
3. The sock must be pulled smoothly over the stump. It may be difficult not to wrinkle the below-knee bandage (Fig. 5.8B).
4. With the prosthetic knee joint locked in full extension and the front fastening fully opened, the temporary prosthesis should be eased up over the stump. The below-knee stump should fit into the felt socket and the prosthetic knee joint should be 1.5 cm above the patient's knee joint (Fig. 5.8C).
5. If there is a rigid pelvic band this should then be fastened (Fig. 5.8D).
6. The front of the leather socket should be fastened correctly (see Fig. 5.8E).

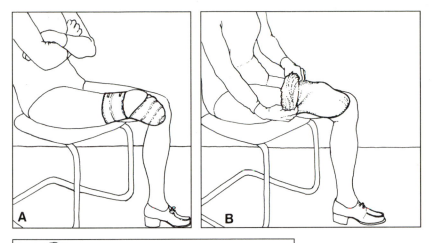

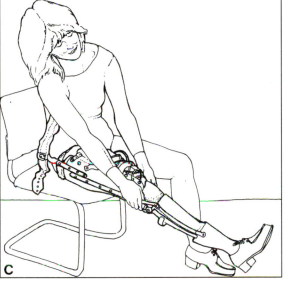

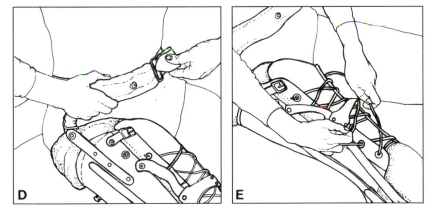

Fig. 5.8 Application of the above-knee/below-knee temporary prosthesis.

7. Any further auxiliary suspension should be fastened and adjusted when the patient is standing.
8. The stump sock should be pulled up over the rim of the socket.

Removal

1. The patient should sit down on a firm surface.
2. The auxiliary suspension should be undone.
3. With the temporary prosthesis locked in extension, the front fastening of the leather socket should be undone completely and the stump eased out of the prosthesis. The patient must maintain the knee joint in full extension throughout this manoeuvre.
4. The stump sock should be pulled off.
5. The bandage should be removed and the skin of the stump checked for any redness or rubbing; occasionally the dressing over the wound may need to be replaced after a period of walking training. The bandage must be replaced.
6. The skin of the thigh should be checked for areas of redness, rubbing or spots.

Dressing

The same method is used as for the above-knee prosthesis. The trouser leg width nearly always has to be widened, as the prosthetic knee and felt socket are very bulky.

Toilet

The same points apply for this prosthesis as for the above-knee prosthesis (see Ch. 11).

Gait re-education

As there is a long lever controlling the prosthesis, there is often a tendency to take too long a stride and to circumduct during the swing phase, instead of hip hitching. The same method of gait re-education is taught as for above-knee prosthesis (see Ch. 11).

The knee joint must be mobilised, and the quadriceps muscle strengthened, with an exercise programme while this temporary stiff knee prosthesis is being used, otherwise transition later on to a patellar tendon bearing prosthesis will be very difficult.

REFERENCES

Abel E W, Frank T G 1991 The design of attendant propelled wheelchairs. Prosthetics and Orthotics International 15(1): 38–45

Alexander A 1971 Immediate postsurgical prosthetic fitting: the role of the physical therapist. Physical Therapy 51(2): 152–157

Bonner F J, Green R F 1982 Pneumatic airleg prosthesis: report of 200 cases. Archives of Physical Medicine and Rehabilitation 63: 383–385

Booker H, Smith S 1988 The AK/BK revisited. Physiotherapy 74(8): 366–368

Burgess E M, Zettl J H 1969 Immediate application of prostheses for amputations. In: Cooper P (ed) Surgery annual. Appleton-Century-Crofts Educational Division. Meredith Corporation, p 371–390

Dickstein R, Pillar T, Mannheim M 1982 The pneumatic post-amputation mobility aid in geriatric rehabilitation. Scandinavian Journal of Rehabilitation Medicine 14: 149–150

Donn J 1991 Use of the TES Belt as an alternative means of suspension with the Ppam Aid. Physiotherapy 77(9): 591–592

Liedberg E, Hommerberg H, Persson B M 1983 Tolerance of early walking with total contact among below-knee amputees — a randomized test. Prosthetics and Orthotics International 7: 91–95

Little J M 1971 A pneumatic weight-bearing temporary prosthesis for below-knee amputees. Lancet 6 Feb: 271–273

McLaurin C A, Brubaker C E 1991 Biomechanics and the wheelchair. Prosthetics and Orthotics International 15(1): 24–37

Monga T N, Symington D C 1984 The airsplint as a pneumatic prosthesis in management of the elderly amputee. Physiotherapy Canada 36(2): 61–65

Parry M, Morrison J D 1989 Use of the Femurett adjustable prosthesis in the assessment and walking training of new above-knee amputees. Prosthetics and Orthotics International 13: 36–38

Ramsey E M 1988 A clinical evaluation of the LIC Femurett as an early training device for the primary above-knee amputee. Physiotherapy 74(12): 598–601

Redhead R G, Davis B C, Robinson K P, Vitali M 1978 Post-amputation pneumatic walking aid. British Journal of Surgery 65(9): 611–612

Van Ross E 1991 Pushchairs. Prosthetics and Orthotics International 15(1): 46–50

6. Assessment for prosthetic rehabilitation

There are different reasons why a primary amputee may be referred to the local prosthetic assessment team:

a. For consultation as to the patient's suitability and readiness for prosthetic rehabilitation. This is the most common reason for referral.

b. For the patient to have an opportunity to see prostheses and, by meeting other amputees, fully understand the implications of learning to use a prosthesis. This is most useful for patients from hospitals where few amputations are performed.

c. For cast or measurement, fitting and subsequent delivery of the prosthesis.

Not every patient referred to the prosthetic rehabilitation team will be fitted with a prosthesis. If the patient is not accepted for prosthetic rehabilitation at the first visit, it must be remembered that this decision can be altered at a later date.

Early referral to the team is needed for patients making an uneventful recovery from surgery. Referral can be made before removal of the sutures. Delay in referral causes an unnecessary postponement of the delivery of the prosthesis.

Later referral to the team is more advisable for the frail and for those with numerous medical complications or multiple physical problems. The patient must be sufficiently fit to endure an ambulance journey to the centre, the somewhat exhausting day seeing unfamiliar faces and the journey home. This type of patient must be able to cope with a full day's rehabilitation programme in hospital.

FACTORS INFLUENCING THE DECISION FOR REFERRAL

1. Does the patient want to walk?

Does the patient fully understand the procedures involved and the amount of personal effort required in prosthetic rehabilitation? If so, then referral must be made.

2. Will it be possible for the patient to walk?

In assessing the patient's potential for prosthetic mobility, the physiotherapist has the following guidelines.

The patient must:

— Be independent transferring
— Be independent dressing
— Have sufficient manual dexterity to manage buckles and buttons
— Have adequate eyesight (blindness alone is not a contra-indication)
— Be able to understand and remember instructions
— Have adequate oxygen perfusion for the increased energy consumption needed for walking with a prosthesis (see Ch. 8).

If patients are unable to demonstrate these basic abilities it is unlikely that they will benefit from prosthetic rehabilitation.

3. Where will the patient walk — who will help?

The patient's accommodation and the help available must be considered. An early home visit will help to ensure that a realistic rehabilitation goal is set, whether this entails supply of a prosthesis, crutches or wheelchair; the visit will also establish whether relatives, friends or neighbours are willing to give encouragement and support. Bilateral amputees may have insufficient room to walk with aids around furniture in their home.

It has been found that amputees who live in either local authority Part III accommodation or continuing care hospitals are most unlikely to use prostheses even if they are supplied, as mobility is safer and faster in a wheelchair.

Younger homeless people will find hostel accommodation easier if they are independent walking, even if the method used is unconventional.

4. Will prosthetic rehabilitation improve the patient's quality of life?

Some patients will be suffering from progressive disease: the stage of the disease must be identified and the prognosis considered in depth. Prosthetic rehabilitation for some is a lengthy, tiring procedure and the benefits of the eventual outcome must be considered.

PROCEDURE OF ASSESSMENT

Written referral is made to the prosthetic rehabilitation team, to whom the hospital notes must be available.

There are now local arrangements throughout the UK for prosthetic referral, which take different forms.

1. To a regional disability services centre (DSC)

The patient travels from the hospital to the centre and is examined by the primary referral team. This team can consist of the following:

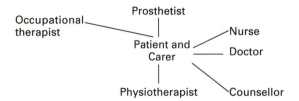

The carer can be either a relative, or a member of staff who has been caring for the patient, or both. Written assessments from the hospital's nurse, physiotherapist, occupational therapist and social worker must be taken along at the first visit.

At Roehampton and other centres, a summary of the assessment and decision made is returned with the patient so that the hospital team remains fully informed.

2. To a satellite DSC clinic within the local district

A doctor and prosthetist can visit locally from the regional DSC, to see all patients referred from the locality. There is a consulting room and workshop facility permanently available. The hospital team are therefore in closer contact and the service is integral to the total care in the district. This type of service improves the access for patients and avoids lengthy tiring journeys, and greater continuity of care can be achieved.

3. Visiting team to the hospital

In some areas there are arrangements whereby a doctor and prosthetist can visit a patient in their hospital ward. This is particularly useful pre-operatively, when the patient may be very sick or infectious, and when an expert opinion on the level of amputation is needed.

Whatever local arrangement is in place, successful referral and rehabilitation will only occur if there is good communication between all involved. The hospital physiotherapist should make every effort to meet all the team members in order to facilitate subsequent telephone or written communication.

PROSTHETIC CONSIDERATIONS OF THE VARIOUS LEVELS OF AMPUTATION

1. Below-knee

Almost all patients with below-knee amputation can be successfully rehabilitated. Many of these patients can manage without walking aids eventually, and should achieve a normal gait pattern. Age is not a contraindication (see Ch. 13).

2. Through- and above-knee

Lack of the natural knee joint requires complex prosthetic replacement which cannot totally replace the natural knee function. Therefore the gait can be slow, and there is a high energy consumption, particularly if the patient has to walk with a stiff knee gait. Younger and fitter patients will use a free knee gait and should walk well without aids eventually (see Chs 11 and 12).

3. Hemipelvectomy and hip disarticulation

The majority of these patients are young and have normal musculature and balance. Therefore they are able to manage the large, complicated prosthesis, coping with prosthetic hip and knee joints. A few patients require a walking aid (see Ch. 10).

4. Bilateral amputees

All these patients must have their accommodation made suitable for wheelchair mobility before referral to the DSC.

All bilateral amputees must understand that prosthetic rehabilitation takes a long time and occurs in stages: great motivation and determination are essential. Initially, temporary prostheses are supplied which are very short and simple; the patient may be half natural height (see Ch. 16). If patients demonstrate that they can cope at home on these temporary prostheses, they are then fitted with modular assembly prostheses which are as short as the component parts technically permit. Their height can be raised later if stamina and ability permits, but even then patients are likely to be several inches shorter than their natural height. Most bilateral amputees will walk with two walking aids, and the hands are therefore not free to carry anything. This limits function.

Energy expenditure both for application of prostheses and walking is enormous, and above average upper limb strength must be present. Patients must be able to lift their body weight using push-up blocks (see Fig. 4.2), and much will depend upon their build and weight.

The presence of knee joints is a vital consideration, as illustrated in the following:

a. The majority of bilateral below-knee amputees will manage prostheses.

b. If there is only one knee joint present, and the contralateral side shows no fixed hip flexion contracture, then prosthetic rehabilitation is possible.

c. Where no natural knee joints remain, prosthetic use is difficult, particularly if there are fixed hip flexion contractures, and if the patient is obese. For the elderly, the wheelchair will be their main means of mobility.

Bilateral above-knee amputees who are not suitable for prosthetic rehabilitation can be supplied with cosmetic prostheses which are for wheelchair use only (see Fig. 6.1). These are of great psychological benefit to both the patient and relatives as the complete body image is maintained. Some patients and physiotherapists, unaware of this option, may strive towards the definitive prosthetic stage solely for the cosmetic benefit and not for mobility (Ch. 16).

5. Upper and lower limb combination

If there is one upper limb and one lower limb amputation present, the artificial leg is usually fitted first and the patient taught to walk. Exercise to the upper limb stump and general postural correction take place while the leg prosthesis is being fitted and delivered. The upper limb prosthesis is supplied afterwards.

If there is one upper limb and bilateral lower limb amputations, it is usual for the upper limb prosthesis to be fitted first. Functional activities from the wheelchair are then achieved. Lower limb exercises and balance training continue while this is taking place and the prostheses for the lower limbs are supplied subsequently.

All these patients face a complicated prosthetic future and it is very important that they are referred to a DSC where there are full prosthetic and rehabilitation facilities.

FOLLOW-UP

It is important that patients are monitored at home following discharge from hospital. The community physiotherapist, local authority occupational therapist, outreach teams, district nurse and GP are in the best position to carry this out. Feedback from these professionals to the DSC doctor is essential and welcomed. Many small problems can occur in the first few weeks, such as alteration in stump volume, inability to operate joint mechanisms, uncertainty regarding social services or benefits, uncertainty as to how to increase and progress activity, and natural anxieties or depression which

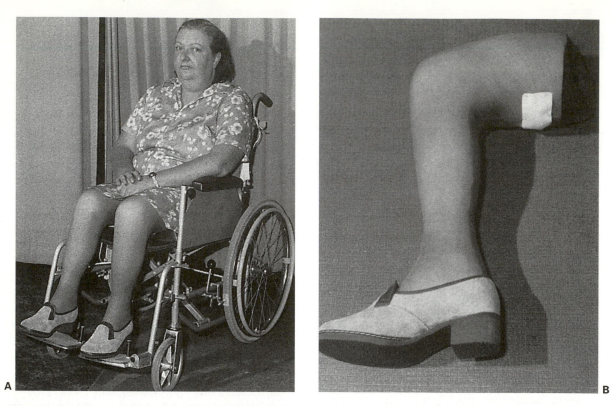

Fig. 6.1 Cosmetic prostheses: (A) a bilateral above-knee amputee wearing cosmetic prostheses; (B) a cosmetic prosthesis with Velcro fastening for attachment to the wheelchair seat.

can occur after leaving a supportive environment. Very often these small issues, if not picked up quickly, can lead to lack of use of the prosthesis. Some centres have an automatic follow-up system but others will need active feedback from patients or carers.

As the months go by, the need for retraining in domestic or leisure activities should be assessed, and the prosthetic prescription may need reviewing. When patients have contacted self-help groups and/or sports or leisure organisations, they may have identified new areas of interest and need in their lives.

Follow-up assessments for the elderly may reveal that:

a. The patient's needs have altered, e.g. change in body weight, loss of other leg or other physical deterioration, change in accommodation, a top-up programme of treatment with physiotherapy and occupational therapy is required.

b. The elderly patient may benefit from the

above in the local geriatric day hospital where full facilities for assessment of medical, physical and social problems are available.

c. The patient may respond to the company and more lively environment of the local day centre or lunch club.

d. The patient may need to give up using prostheses and require help in achieving other forms of mobility for an independent existence.

OTHER FORMS OF MOBILITY

1. Wheelchair (see Ch. 5)

It is likely that the patient has already been supplied with a wheelchair, but if it was thought that the chair would only be used occasionally and that most of the time the patient would walk, then reassessment must take place. The size and type of chair, its condition and the type of cushion used must be checked to ensure maximum comfort. The home environment must be visited to assess access, transfer heights and toilet and bathing facilities.

2. Hopping

Some patients may be able to hop with either crutches or a frame sufficiently well to move around the home. This form of mobility may have to be explored in combination with the wheelchair as some rooms may be inaccessible with the chair and structural alterations inadvisable or impossible.

Occasionally, hopping may be considered by the patient to be faster and easier than using a prosthesis, particularly for those with a painful stump or high level of amputation.

3. Walking directly on weightbearing stumps

The Symes and through-knee levels are ideal for this. Some form of stump cover should be supplied (see Fig. 6.2), Some below-knee amputees may walk around on their hands and knees.

4. Other ideas

Occasionally the physiotherapist must devise another system of mobility. For example, there was an elderly bilateral above-knee amputee who found prosthetic rehabilitation impossible. His wheelchair could not be used in his flat where he lived with his daughter and grandchildren. He did not wish to move from this happy family environment so a low platform on castors was made for him to scoot around on. It was checked that his upper limb strength was sufficient for him to transfer both down to this board and back up again in stages (see Fig. 6.3).

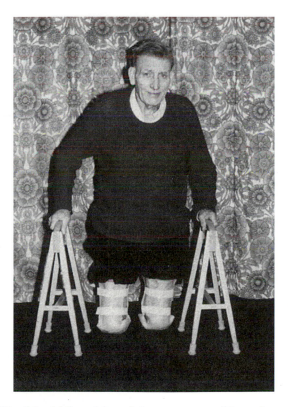

Fig. 6.2 A bilateral through-knee amputee walking, using stump covers made of Plastazote lined with Velvetex and fastened with Velcro.

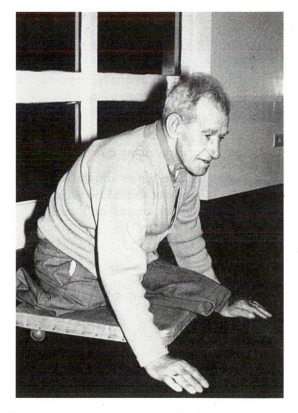

Fig. 6.3 An alternative to a wheelchair for a bilateral amputee.

REFERENCES

Buttenshaw P J 1991 The multidisciplinary team approach for the assessment of primary amputees. Personal communication

Chilvers A S, Browse N L 1971 The social fate of the amputee. Lancet 27 Nov: 1192–1193, 1315–1316

Doherty S M, Nichols P J R 1974 Non-prosthetic problems of rehabilitation of the ischaemic lower limb amputee. Orthopaedics 7(2): 77–85

Hamilton A 1981 Rehabilitation of the leg amputee in the community. Journal of Postgraduate Medicine 225: 1487–1497

Hamilton A, Williams E, Nichols P J R 1974 The elderly lower limb amputee. Update 9: 1641–1650

Hamilton E A, Nichols P J R 1972 Rehabilitation of the elderly lower-limb amputee. British Medical Journal 2: 95–99

Hanspal R S, Fisher K 1991 Assessment of cognitive and psychomotor function and rehabilitation of elderly people with prostheses. British Medical Journal 302: 940

Holden J M, Fernie G R 1987 Extent of artificial limb use following rehabilitation. Journal of Orthopaedic Research 5: 562–568

Hubbard W A 1989 Rehabilitation outcomes for elderly lower limb amputees. Australian Journal of Physiotherapy 35(4): 219–224

Jain S K 1988 Rehabilitation of elderly amputees. Armed Forces Medical Journal India 44(1): 15–20

Kay J 1991 Domiciliary rehabilitation of elderly amputees. Physiotherapy 77 (1): 60–61.

Narang I C, Mathur B P, Singh P, Jape V S 1984 Functional capabilities of lower limb amputees. Prosthetics and Orthotics International 8: 43–51

Parish J G, James D W 1982 A method for evaluating the level of independence during the rehabilitation of the disabled. Rheumatology and Rehabilitation 21: 107–114

Siriwardena G J A, Bertrand P V 1991 Factors influencing rehabilitation of arteriosclerotic lower limb amputees. Journal of Rehabilitation Research and Development 28(3): 35–44

7. Prosthetic services for the amputee

HISTORY

A service for the supply of artificial limbs to members of the armed forces was started in 1915 when the owner of Roehampton House gave it to the nation for use as a convalescent home for war wounded, especially amputees. This was followed by the setting up of facilities in other parts of the country, and by 1918 the first Director of Artificial Limb Supplies was appointed by the Minister of Pensions. During the Second World War there was a further influx of patients but the service still existed predominately for war injuries until the inception of the British National Health Service (NHS) in 1948. The system then expanded to take in civilian amputees as well as the ex-servicemen already under its care.

The supply of artificial limbs then became the responsibility of central government through the Department of Health and Social Security (DHSS) Artificial Limb Service. There were about 30 centres throughout England and Wales supplying services, including some smaller satellite centres. The main centres also provided a wheelchair and small surgical supply service. These centres were known as Artificial Limb and Appliance Centres (ALACs).

The organisation of the Scottish prosthetic services became the responsibility of the NHS and is administered by the Scottish Home and Health Department; the local prosthetic services are operated by the Health Authority Boards. At present there are six centres, two in Glasgow and one each in Edinburgh, Dundee, Aberdeen and Inverness. Prosthetic services (including components used) are the subject of contracts negotiated locally (e.g. regionally or area-wide).

In May 1984, a group was set up 'to review and report on the adequacy, quality and management of the various services received by patients in Artificial Limb and Appliance Centres (ALACs) in England, on the respective roles of the staff of the centres and the NHS, and commercial manufacturers, having regard to the need to promote efficiency and cost effectiveness'. The group was chaired by Professor Ian McColl, now Lord McColl of Dulwich. It recommended changes in:

— The organisation and management of the Artificial Limb Service and Wheelchair Service
— War Pensioner's Appliances and Invalid Vehicle Services.

To enable these changes a special health authority, the Disablement Services Authority (DSA), was created in 1987 as a transitional management medium to adopt certain strategic aims covering:

— improved management of human resources, for the wheelchair and artificial limb service
— provision of services with the maximum of efficiency, economy and effectiveness, recognising quality issues
— improved communications and commitment
— integration of the total service into the NHS by 1 April 1991.

THE PRESENT

The wheelchair service is now the responsibility of every district health authority, each having its own local arrangements for assessment, delivery and after-service.

The supply of artificial limbs is based on the regional Disablement Services Centres (DSCs), incorporating the services of multidisciplinary teams, e.g. consultant in rehabilitation medicine, prosthetist, occupational therapists, physiotherapists and nursing staff. In some areas satellite centres or district general hospitals will supply these services. Much depends on local policies and strategies.

Clinical audit exists throughout the regions and budgeting and financial issues are being monitored using the agreed performance indicators. Quality measures are set up across the whole service, which is now fully integrated in the NHS. Funding was 'ring fenced' for 2 years after integration into the NHS to permit a stable situation whilst provider/purchaser arrangements were set up in line with the NHS reforms.

PROSTHETIC SERVICES

The prosthetic service to the patient is independent from the manufacturing companies producing hardware and components. Independent prosthetic services are able to assess, fit and deliver a variety of prosthetic components produced by different manufacturers. A flexible prosthetic service can be found throughout the country using components from different companies. This permits a wide choice for the amputee's individual needs. Contracts for prosthetic services are tendered for every 3 years, promoting competition.

At present all components have to comply with standards set by the British Standards Institution and the Consumer Protection Act and standards set down by BS5750. It is envisaged that EC legislation will gradually introduce new markets which should enable greater choice of artificial limbs and components for the consumer. Great emphasis, however, will be given to quality and safety.

As the prosthetic service has now been devolved down to regional, and in some cases district, localities, quality and cost will have to be carefully monitored to ensure that the advantages of supplying a flexible service are not denigrated by poor standards of care.

Referral to prosthetic services

The hospital rehabilitation team will refer the primary amputee to the DSC rehabilitation team. This referral must include diagnosis, date of operation, surgical techniques and details of the physical ability of the amputee, and a rehabilitation assessment. Information on social circumstances covering the type of accommodation and support available to the amputee on discharge is also invaluable.

At Roehampton DSC, special referral forms have been agreed between the DSC and referring district general hospitals and relate to physiotherapy, occupational therapy, social and nursing details. There are also contact names supplied for the DSC rehabilitation team to use if further details are required. Communications between all staff are absolutely vital.

The DSC team, which includes the prosthetist, will decide on the needs of the amputee and the type of prostheses necessary. Following consultation with the patient and the carer the final prescription of the prosthesis will then be decided.

The prosthetist will make a plaster-of-Paris cast of the stump for the socket, explaining both the casting, fitting and delivery procedures, and will demonstrate to the amputee a complete prosthesis. It will be the prosthetist's decision, in discussion with the team, to select the various components available from the component manufacturers.

The amputee will return to the prosthetist for a fitting of the socket. If this is comfortable the components will be added and standing and walking practice will be possible in the parallel bars. During this time the prosthetist will adjust the components to ensure correct static and dynamic alignment. This takes time and patience especially for those who may be elderly and frail or have multiple injuries.

In some cases, where the stump is fluctuating in volume or there are several medical problems, it may be necessary for the amputee to attend a second fitting. This can be extremely disappointing and reasons for these problems should be fully explained. The prosthetist may well request some physiotherapy sessions using the prosthesis in an unfinished state, observe the gait pattern and make minor adjustments from day to day so that maximum comfort and optimum alignment are attained.

At Roehampton DSC the amputee will attend the physiotherapy department for several sessions following the fitting of the prosthesis. This enables the physiotherapist to commence gait re-education and the prosthetist to monitor the alignment and comfort of the prosthesis. Once this is achieved the prosthesis is covered with its cosmesis and the amputee usually returns to the referring hospital's out-patient department for further prosthetic rehabilitation.

When the amputee, prosthetist and doctor are satisfied with the prescription, fit, function and cosmesis of the prosthesis, delivery is taken and referral for further rehabilitation is made. The prosthetist will have explained and instructed the amputee in the basic principles of the prosthesis.

The prosthetist will issue the correct size of stump sock. A note of the size is made on the amputee's record card and retained. Stump socks can be made of:

a. Wool mix. This is the thickest material obtainable; it protects the skin and absorbs perspiration.

b. Cotton mix. This is normally thinner. Three thin cotton socks are equal to the thickness of one woollen sock. There are also brushed cotton socks which are of a similar thickness to the woollen socks.

c. Nylon. This is a very thin covering which reduces the friction of the socket against the skin but takes up so little room in the socket that it should not be regarded as padding.

Information on the care of socks and their specific use should be given immediately by the prosthetist. Most DSCs supply information leaflets (see Ch. 18). It is also possible to purchase special socks, and some established amputees with specific problems find this useful. At present there are several different types and combinations of materials for stump socks on trial.

It is crucial that the physiotherapist, the prosthetist and the doctor are in close communication during the early stages of prosthetic rehabilitation. In many cases, especially with the modular prosthesis where the cosmetic foam encases the components, it is impossible to ascertain the exact functional ability of various components by observation only. The physiotherapist must ensure that specific details of the prosthesis are known and understood and should not rely on information passed on by the amputee.

The physiotherapist must examine the whole prosthesis: the socket, suspension, alignment and components. Both static and dynamic alignments must be checked, with special reference to the type of shoes worn. Footwear and heel height will alter the alignment of the prosthesis which in turn may affect the lumbar spine. This will cause pain and musculoskeletal problems and often have a direct relation on the amputee's functional ability in using the prosthesis (see Ch. 9).

It is important that the physiotherapist understands the different components available and their suitability for each amputee. The components can be changed if necessary, but this must be a team decision. The physiotherapist must remain in contact with the doctor and the prosthetist to ensure that, if alterations are to be made, they are correct, and that appropriate training and education is given to the amputee.

PROSTHETIC CONSTRUCTION

All prostheses have the following features:

1. A prosthetic socket to contain the stump and provide for weightbearing and stability
2. Some form of suspension, either by socket design or additional straps
3. Prosthetic joints and interjoint segments to replace those amputated
4. A base for contact with the floor.

The majority of prostheses supplied are of endoskeletal design, the supporting structure being housed within a soft cosmetic covering. These prostheses can incorporate a variety of components to suit the needs of the individual amputee (Fig. 7.1).

The components can be interchangeable and this can be achieved during a day's visit to the prosthetist. An example of this would be a patient changing the knee component from a locking knee to a free knee gait using swing phase controls.

The endoskeletal prostheses have a foam covering to give as natural an appearance as possible, and every effort is made to achieve cosmetic acceptability for the amputee (see Fig. 7.2).

There is still a demand, however, for the conventional prostheses which are of exoskeletal design. Unlike the endoskeletal prostheses, the outside shell is the supporting structure. These prostheses are less adjustable in that the variety of components available cannot be housed within their construction, nor can change of prescription be quickly achieved. They are, however, still useful for limited overseas supply, being of a simple and sturdy construction. Also, they are still popular with many experienced and older limb wearers who do not wish to alter their prosthetic design.

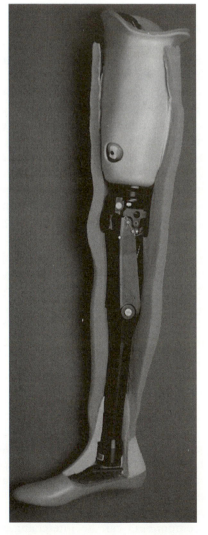

Fig. 7.1 A modular prosthesis for an above-knee amputation demonstrating the various components within the cosmetic foam covering. (Reproduced from Redhead et al 1991.)

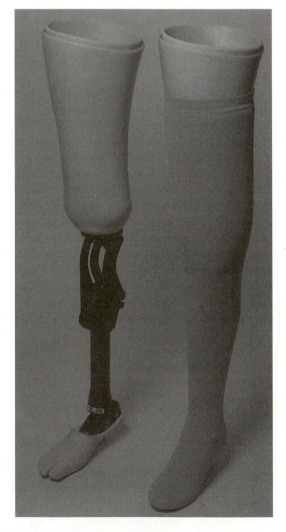

Fig. 7.2 The Endolite prosthesis for the through-knee amputee. It has a four-bar linkage knee mechanism and a multiflex ankle mechanism. (Photograph by kind permission of C. A. Blatchford & Sons Ltd.)

Materials used

Thermoplastics

The majority of prosthetic sockets are fabricated from these materials, e.g. polypropylene. There are also plastic materials which are more pliable and can be used as inner sockets for some difficult above-knee fittings, e.g. Surlyn. The Icelandic–Swedish–New York (ISNY) socket is an example of the use of these flexible plastics (see Fig. 7.3) which permits a pliability that enhances both suspension and comfort for the above knee amputee.

Some translucent materials can also be used for check sockets for particularly difficult fittings to enable the prosthetist to ensure the correct fit.

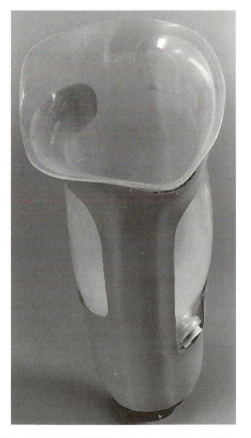

Fig. 7.3 A left-sided ISNY socket (medial view). The carbon fibre reinforced medial strut carries the load, and the flexible inner liner is supported on two wings from the top of the strut. (Photograph by kind permission of C. A. Blatchford & Sons Ltd.)

Silicones

Silicone rubber materials are very soft and are used for suspension sockets and cosmetic restoration.

Foam

The majority of endoskeletal prostheses are clad in a cosmetic foam. This is skilfully fashioned to give an excellent cosmetic appearance as well as protecting the components. Much of this foam has a memory molecular composition ensuring that after compression, e.g. full knee flexion, the material returns to its original shape. Other thermoplastic foams are used for socket linings, e.g. P E Lite (see Ch. 13).

Carbon fibre

This medium is used extensively in the components and supporting structures for endoskeletal prostheses. It permits strength with light weight, which is ideal for the amputee, both for function and reduced energy consumption.

Metal

This is used for some sockets and the outside shell of exoskeletal prostheses. The metal used is generally Duralumin, an aluminium alloy. Steel and other alloys are used in some components, especially knee mechanisms. Some primary amputees are supplied initially with metal sockets as metal can be an adjustable medium for the prosthetist when dealing with a stump fluctuating in size.

Leather

This is still used as a soft medium for suspension straps and linings, or it can be stiffened (blocked) for some sockets and thigh corsets (see Ch. 5).

Wood

This was extensively used for fashioning prostheses in the past, but is rare now in the UK. However, it is still a useful material for some overseas amputees and is particularly valuable for those living in hot humid climates, as the skin of the stump is more comfortable and able to breathe. Some wood fabrication may still be seen in prosthetic feet.

Examples of different prosthetic components

In Chapters 10–14 some of the more commonly available components and construction methods will be briefly identified. These are constantly being upgraded and altered to keep pace with the needs of the amputee. The availability and variety of prescription are illustrated below, using prosthetic feet as an example.

SACH (solid ankle cushioned heel) foot

This is a simple foot with no ankle joint. The plastic foam of the foot has a wedge section in the heel which may be varied in density to suit the weight and activity of the amputee. This wedge absorbs the shock load at heel strike and simulates ankle movement. At toe off the material used in the construction of the foot enables flexion to occur in the forefoot (see Fig. 7.4).

Uniaxial ankles

Here there is ankle movement which is commonly controlled by two rubber bumpers, one of which controls plantar flexion on heel strike and the other dorsiflexion during the last stages of the stance phase. The foot can be made of wood covered with leather, but is more likely to be plastic moulded. The construction of a wooden forefoot permits flexion at toe off (see Fig. 7.5).

Multiaxial ankles

The construction of these components enables a complete range of movements, i.e. plantar flexion, dorsiflexion, inversion and eversion, and also rotation. These can be adjusted for each amputee's need, weight and activity level by increasing or decreasing the hardness of the rubber component and snubber in the ankle mechanism (see Fig. 7.6). The keel of the foot is carbon fibre reinforced plastic.

Energy-storing prosthetic feet

Some examples of energy conserving, or dynamic elastic response (DER) feet are the Seattle Light Foot, the Quantum Foot and the Springlite Foot (see Figs 7.7 and 7.8). The design of these feet gives a smooth, easy gait pattern for the amputee.

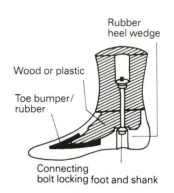

Fig. 7.4 A cross-section of the SACH foot.

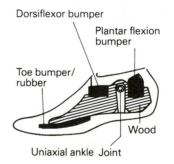

Fig. 7.5 A cross-section of the uniaxial foot.

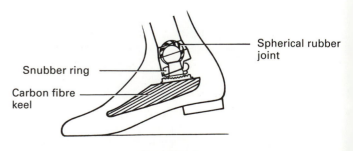

Fig. 7.6 The multiaxial ankle.

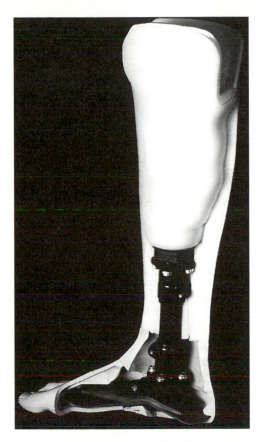

Fig. 7.7 A below-knee prosthesis with a Quantum foot. (Photograph by kind permission of Vessa Ltd.)

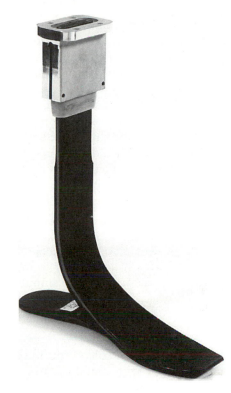

Fig. 7.8 The Springlite Foot. (Photograph by kind permission of Springlite Manufacturing, Utah.)

The energy-storing capacity enables some amputees to be able to jump and run. These feet contain a springy component which compresses with weightbearing. The energy thus stored is released during the last stages of the stance phase and propels the prosthesis forwards, giving an extra spring action at push off. These feet are suitable for most endoskeletal and exoskeletal prostheses.

These are just examples of prosthetic feet that are available. There are many more with specific designs and variations. Some feet have the added adjustability in that the heel height can be altered by approximately 2 cm. This enables the amputee to wear shoes of different heel heights. Some prosthetic feet can be adjusted by the amputee, others have to be altered by the prosthetist (see Fig. 7.9).

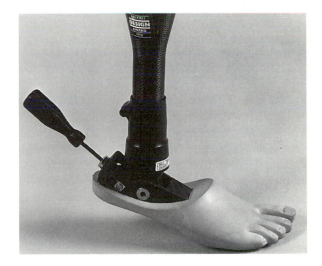

Fig. 7.9 The multiflex ankle mechanism showing the heel height adjustment. (Photograph by kind permission of C. A. Blatchford & Sons Ltd.)

RESEARCH AND DEVELOPMENT

There is considerable research and development in the field of prosthetics. The desire to improve function, comfort and cosmetic appearance combined with reduced energy consumption is on-going.

Computerisation of the fabrication of sockets has met with some success. Computer-aided design and computer-aided manufacture (CAT-CAM) are now being introduced on a limited basis. These methods may make it possible to reproduce a socket of constant size and consistent quality. A variety of new components, permitting kneeling, sitting crossed legged, etc, have also been developed.

The process of developing and designing new components and ideas will continue to meet the on-going needs and demands of the amputee.

CURRENT AWARENESS

It is important for those physiotherapists who are directly involved with amputees to keep up to date with all the new available hardware.

Prosthetic design and manufacture is constantly changing and this will increase as the European and world markets become accessible.

The International Society of Prosthetics and Orthotics (ISPO) is the most relevant organisation with which to be in touch. The UK has a strong member branch. The Society supplies the international journal and newsletter; both provide valuable reading in research and good practice.

Each year there is as annual scientific meeting for the presentation of research and exchange of information. Every 3 years there is an international conference with participants coming from all over the world. In some areas of the UK therapy networks exist.

Clinical audit, which is already set up in the DSCs, is another way of both learning and improving quality. Physiotherapists must be included in these initiatives using their national and local standards of practice and initiate their own evaluation of outcome and treatment modalities. This should involve formal research.

A bibliography of some relevant literature can be found in the Appendix.

REFERENCES

Buttenshaw P 1991 Amputees benefit from teamwork. Therapy Weekly 17(41): 2

Canby T Y 1989 Reshaping our lives. National Geographic 176(6): 746–760

English A W G, Gregory Dean A A 1980 The artificial limb service. Health Trends 12: 77

Fernie G R, Halsall A P, Ruder K 1984 Shape sensing as an educational aid for student prosthetists. Prosthetics and Orthotics International 8: 87–90

Fillauer C E, Pritham C H, Fillauer K D 1989 Evolution and development of the silicone suction socket (3S) for below-knee prostheses. Journal of Prosthetics and Orthotics 1(2): 92–103

Foort J 1979 Modular prosthetics — a philosophical view. Prosthetics and Orthotics International 3: 140–143

Hirons R R 1991 The prosthetic treatment of lower limb deficiency. Prosthetics and Orthotics International 15: 112–116

Hughes J 1978 Education in prosthetics and orthotics. Prosthetics and Orthotics International 2: 51–53

Kabra S G, Narayanan R 1991 Ankle-foot prosthesis with articulated human bone endoskeleton: force-deflection and fatigue study. Journal of Rehabilitation Research and Development 28(3): 13–22

Limb M, Calnan M 1990 Artificial limbs: a real need. Health Service Journal 100(15 Nov) 5227: 1696–1697

Menard M R, McBride M E, Sanderson D J, Murray D D 1992 Comparative biomechanical analysis of energy-storing prosthetic feet. Archives of Physical Medicine and Rehabilitation 73(5): 451–458

Mensch G 1986 Aids and equipment. Prosthetic update. Physiotherapy Canada 38(6): 369–371

Michael J W 1992 Prosthetic feet: options for the older client. Topics in Geriatric Rehabilitation 8(1): 30–38

Murphy E F 1984 Sockets, linings and interfaces. Clinical Prosthetics and Orthotics 8(3): 4–10

Nielsen C C 1991 A survey of amputees: functional level and life satisfaction, information needs and the prosthetist's role. Journal of Prosthetics and Orthotics 3(3): 125–129

Redhead R G et al 1991 Prescribing lower limb prostheses. DSA ISBN 0-9517249-0-8

Royal College of Physicians 1986 Physical disability and beyond. Reprinted from Journal of The Royal College of Physicians of London 20(3) (complete report)

Southwell M 1983 The history and design development of artificial limbs. Thesis, Department of Industrial Design, Manchester Polytechnic

Taylor J S 1979 Modular assembly above-knee prostheses. Prosthetics and Orthotics International 3: 144–146

Topper A K, Fernie G R 1990 An evaluation of computer aided design of below-knee prosthetic sockets. Prosthetics and Orthotics International 14(3): 136–142

Torburn L et al 1990 Below-knee gait with dynamic elastic response prosthetic feet: a pilot study. Journal of Rehabilitation Research and Development 27(4): 369–384

Van Jaarsveld H W L et al 1990 Stiffness and hysteresis properties of some prosthetic feet. Prosthetics and Orthotics International 14(3): 117–124

8. Normal locomotion and prosthetic replacement

Normal human locomotion is the product of many complex interactions between the forces generated within the body and several external forces acting upon it. It has been described as a series of rhythmical, alternating movements of the extremities and trunk which result in the forward movement of the centre of gravity. In this chapter we do not intend to describe locomotion in anything like its actual complexity, but the presentation here of fundamental facts about locomotion should help the reader to understand the gait of the amputee and some aspects of prosthetic design. Gait re-education requires the ability to analyse each phase of the gait cycle with its integrated motions of the various segments of the body. Success relies on the accurate knowledge of the functional characteristics of the normal locomotor system. Considering the complexity of movement in normal locomotion, prosthetic replacement, while not perfect, can be surprisingly good in the lower limb. However, the amputee has to adapt his gait to the individual design, components and alignment of the prosthesis supplied.

THE GAIT CYCLE

A gait cycle consists of the activity which occurs between the heel strike of one leg to the next heel strike of the same leg (Fig. 8.1). The cycle is divided into two phases: the stance phase and the swing phase.

Stance phase

This begins at heel strike on one leg and ends at toe off on the same leg. There are six subdivisions of stance phase:

1. *Heel strike*: the instant the heel touches the ground
2. *Foot flat*: the sole of the foot touches the ground
3. *Mid stance*: the body weight is swung directly over the supporting extremity and continues to rotate over the foot
4. *Heel off*: the heel of the supporting extremity leaves the ground

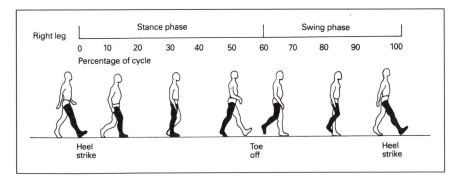

Fig. 8.1 The gait cycle.

5. *Push off*: the body is propelled forwards by the powerful action of the calf muscles
6. *Toe off*: the instant when the toe rises from the ground

Swing phase

This begins where stance phase ends and is the period between toe off of one foot and heel strike of the same foot.

There are three subdivisions of swing phase:

1. *Acceleration*: the instant the toe leaves the ground the leg must be accelerated to overtake the body in preparation for the next heel strike
2. *Mid swing*: this occurs when the swinging leg passes directly beneath the body
3. *Deceleration*: this occurs after mid swing when the forward motion of the leg is restrained to control the position of the foot immediately before heel strike

Stride length is the distance between foot flat to foot flat on the same leg; in normal subjects walking at an average velocity of 2.5 m.p.h. it is 76–81 cm.

Double support

This is the period when both feet are in contact with the ground simultaneously, and occurs between push off and toe off on one foot and heel strike and foot flat on the other. The length of time of the double support period is directly related to cadence (walking speed): as cadence increases the period of double support decreases (and stride length increases). The normal walking speed for an adult male is approximately 96 steps/min. The absence of double support indicates that a person is running rather than walking; in the average adult male this starts at a speed of 140 steps/min.

Time distribution in the gait cycle

At normal walking speeds the stance phase accounts for approximately 60% of the gait cycle, the swing phase for approximately 40% of the cycle, and there is double support for approximately 20% of the cycle.

THE CENTRE OF GRAVITY

The centre of gravity (CG) of the body is an imaginary point at which all the weight of the body may be assumed to be concentrated at a certain instant. Its precise location is not fixed. In the normal body standing erect, its location is slightly anterior to the second sacral vertebra.

Walking may be viewed as the displacement of the body CG from one point to another. To walk with a minimum expenditure of energy it is necessary to minimise variations of the instantaneous velocity of the body CG and the vertical and lateral displacement of the body CG. Changes in velocity and displacement of the CG is work which requires energy. The principal motions and the velocity of the CG in normal walking are determined by a number of observable gait characteristics.

CLINICALLY OBSERVABLE CHARACTERISTICS OF GAIT

Vertical displacement of the body CG
(Fig. 8.2)

In the normal walking pattern, the body CG undergoes a rhythmic upward and downward motion as it moves forward. The highest point occurs when the supporting limb is in mid stance; the lowest point occurs at the time of double support when both feet are in contact with the ground.

The normal vertical displacement of the body CG is approximately 5 cm and the most significant clinically observable factor limiting this excursion is the coordinated function of the knee and ankle. Immediately after heel strike, with the knee fully extended, the knee begins to flex and the ankle

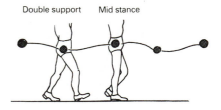

Fig. 8.2 Vertical movement of the CG while walking.

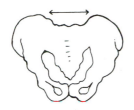

Fig. 8.3   Lateral displacement of the body CG is approx. 5 cm with each stride.

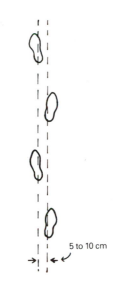

5 to 10 cm

Fig. 8.4   The width of the walking base controls the lateral displacement of the pelvis.

begins to plantar flex. The net result is reduction of the extent to which the CG displaces upwards as the pelvis moves over the support leg. The above-knee amputee walking with a locked knee will therefore display a greater vertical displacement of the body CG, significantly raising the energy cost of walking.

Lateral displacement of the CG (Fig. 8.3)

As weight is transferred from one leg to the other there is a shift of the pelvis and trunk to the weightbearing side. The body CG, as it moves forward, not only undergoes the vertical motion already described, but oscillates from side to side as well.

The normal lateral CG displacement walking on level ground is approximately 5 cm, and there are three clinically observable factors limiting this excursion:

a. Width of the walking base

b. Horizontal dip of the pelvis

c. Transverse rotation of the pelvis.

Width of the walking base (Fig. 8.4)

In normal walking, one foot is placed ahead of the other either side of an imaginary line of progression. If a lines is drawn through successive mid-points of heel strike of each foot, the distance between these parallel lines represents the width of the walking base. In normal subjects this varies between 5 and 10 cm. The lateral displacement of the body CG is such that it remains over the supporting leg. If an amputee walks with an abducted gait the lateral displacement increases and therefore the energy cost increases.

Horizontal dip of the pelvis (Fig. 8.5)

This is the angular motion of the pelvis in the frontal plane. The pelvis tilts at mid stance about 5°, listing downward from the weightbearing limb.

Transverse rotation of the pelvis (Fig. 8.6)

The pelvis appears to rotate about a vertical axis which assists the advancement of one extremity while the other is fixed to the ground. This keeps the width of the walking base within normal limits. The rotation actually occurs at each hip joint, which passes from relative external rotation to relative internal rotation during the stance phase. The femur rotates approximately 10° with respect to the pelvis. The torque transmitted

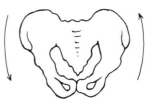

Fig. 8.5   The horizontal dip of the pelvis on the unsupported side is controlled by the hip abductors on the opposite side. This controls lateral displacement of the body CG.

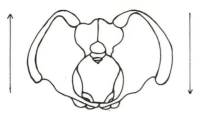

Fig. 8.6 Transverse rotation of the pelvis permits one leg to move forwards while the other is fixed with minimal lateral displacement of the body CG.

through the femur generates a relative rotation of approximately 9° between the femur and the tibia.

Velocity of the body CG

This refers to the instantaneous velocity of the CG, i.e. its velocity at specific instants. This is constantly changing during the gait cycle as weight is applied and removed from each leg.

A normal subject tends to walk at a fairly well-defined average velocity of 2.5 m.p.h. (*Velocity* = step length × no. of steps/min.) It is assumed that this speed represents an optimal velocity at which energy consumption is minimal. One of the most important factors is the weight distribution of the segments of the limb, which at swing phase acts as a pendulum.

If restraints are imposed or abnormal function occurs, changes of the instantaneous velocity of the CG will be necessary to maintain any particular average velocity. The distribution of weight in the leg segments will affect this velocity. Examples of this are a normal subject walking in Wellington boots covered in mud, compared with walking in bare feet, and an above-knee amputee wearing a conventional limb compared with an above-knee amputee wearing a lightweight limb.

Arm swing

Movements of the arm are opposite to the movements of the leg, thus providing opposite reaction forces. Arm movements with trunk rotation allow balance and symmetry of gait. A bilateral arm amputee often experiences gross standing and walking balance problems because of the lack of reciprocal upper trunk movements.

ANALYSIS OF MOTIONS AND FORCES

The pattern of joint motions used in walking minimises the vertical and lateral displacement of the body CG. Human gait is produced by specific motions which occur at the joints and there are forces which produce those motions. These in turn result from the interaction between the internal forces produced inside the body by the muscles, and external forces, principally the influence of gravity.

Before looking at the forces and motions at the major joints during walking, brief explanations of terms and definitions are given to help the reader understand the mechanics of locomotion.

— *Newton's Third Law*: To every action, there is an equal and opposite reaction.
— *Force*: The physical action which tends to change the position of a body in space.
— *Vector*: The graphical representation of a force represented by a line, the length of which is proportional to the magnitude of the force, the direction of which corresponds to that of the force and the start of which represents the points of application of the force.
— *The moment of a force (torque)*: The action of a force producing a tendency for rotation to occur about an axis.
— *Resultant force* (Fig. 8.7): A single force which will produce the same effect as two or more forces; e.g. ground reaction force: this has three components:
  • Vertical force
  • Horizontal force in the line of walking (fore and aft shear)
  • Horizontal force at right angles to the line of walking (lateral shear)
— *Work*: Force × distance moved.
— *Energy*: The capacity to perform work.
— *Efficiency*: The ratio of work done to energy expended

Analysis in the sagittal plane

Heel strike (Fig. 8.8)

— *Ground reaction*:
  Anterior to the hip causing a flexion moment.
  Anterior to the knee causing an extension moment.

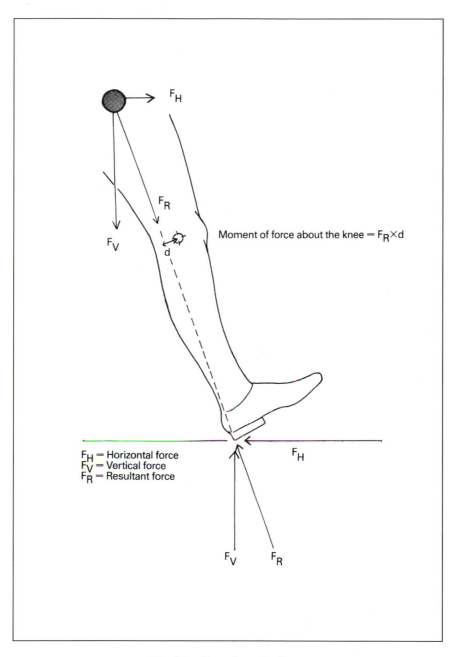

Moment of force about the knee $= F_R \times d$

F_H = Horizontal force
F_V = Vertical force
F_R = Resultant force

Fig. 8.7   Ground reaction force.

Posterior to the ankle causing a plantar flexion moment.

— *The hip* is flexed to 25° and the extensor muscles are active in preventing further flexion.

— *The knee* is in extension at heel strike. The extension moment is overcome by the action of the hamstrings and the knee begins to flex.

— *The ankle* is in the neutral position, then begins to plantar flex. This is controlled by eccentric work in the dorsiflexor muscles.

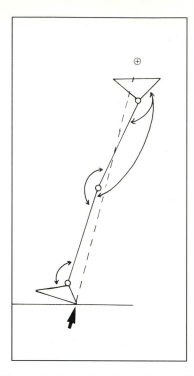

Fig. 8.8 Heel strike. (Reproduced from Hughes J, Jacobs N 1979 Normal human locomotion. Prosthetics and Orthotics International 3: 4–12, by kind permission of the authors and publishers.)

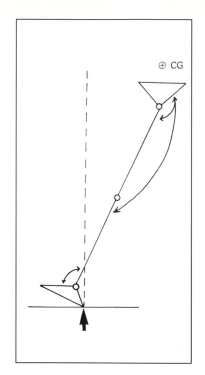

Fig. 8.9 Shortly after heel strike. (Reproduced from Hughes J, Jacobs N 1979 Normal human locomotion. Prosthetics and Orthotics International 3: 4–12, by kind permission of the authors and publishers.)

Shortly after heel strike (Fig. 8.9)

— *Ground reaction*:
  Anterior to the hip causing a flexion moment.
  Posterior to the knee causing flexion moment.
  Posterior to the ankle causing a plantar flexion moment.
— *The hip* is held in 25° of flexion by the controlling action of the extensor muscles preventing excessive flexion.
— *The knee* continues to flex. The rate of flexion is controlled by the quadriceps working eccentrically.
— *The ankle* is in 5° of plantar flexion and continues to plantar flex under the eccentric control of the dorsiflexors.

Foot flat (Fig. 8.10)

— *Ground reaction*:
  Anterior to the hip causing a flexion moment.
  Posterior to the knee causing a flexion moment.

Posterior to the ankle causing a plantar flexion moment.
— *The hip* is in 25° of flexion then begins to extend.
— *The knee* reaches 15° of flexion and continues to flex until it reaches 20° shortly after foot flat. It then begins to extend. The quadriceps muscle controls both of these movements.
— *The ankle* is in 10° of plantar flexion. The plantar flexion moments reduce as the ground reaction line moves along the foot and the dorsiflexor activity diminishes. As the ground reaction passes anterior to the ankle joint the segments of the supporting limb begin to rotate over the fixed foot.

Mid stance (Fig. 8.11)

— *Ground reaction*:
  Passes through the hip joint so no moment is produced.

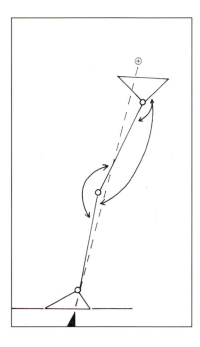

Fig. 8.10   Foot flat. (Reproduced from Hughes J, Jacobs N 1979 Normal human locomotion. Prosthetics and Orthotics International 3: 4–12, by kind permission of the authors and publishers.)

Posterior to the knee causing a flexion moment.
Anterior to the ankle causing a dorsiflexion moment.
— *The hip* is in 10° of flexion and begins to extend as the ground reaction moves posterior to the hip joint shortly after mid stance.
— *The knee* reaches 10° of flexion and continues to extend.
— *The ankle* is in 5° of dorsiflexion and continues to dorsiflex due to ground reaction. This is controlled by the plantar flexors.

Heel off (Fig. 8.12)

— *Ground reactions*:
Posterior to the hip causing an extension moment.
Anterior to the knee causing an extension moment.
Anterior to the ankle causing a dorsiflexion moment.

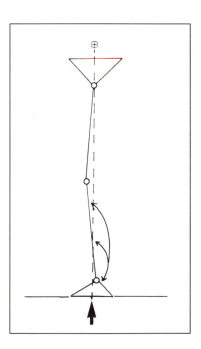

Fig. 8.11   Mid stance. (Reproduced from Hughes J, Jacobs N 1979 Normal human locomotion. Prosthetics and Orthotics International 3: 4–12, by kind permission of the authors and publishers.)

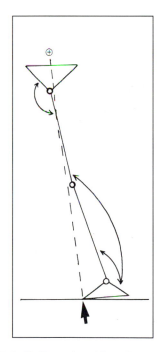

Fig. 8.12   Heel off. (Reproduced from Hughes J, Jacobs N 1979 Normal human locomotion. Prosthetics and Orthotics International 3: 4–12, by kind permission of the authors and publishers.)

— *The hip* reaches full extension then begins to flex controlled by the hip flexors.
— *The knee* is flexed about 2°.
— *The ankle* reaches 15° of dorsiflexion after which it plantar flexes due to a powerful contraction of the calf muscles which counteracts the dorsiflexion moment and assists in propelling the body forward.

Toe off (Fig. 8.13)

— *Ground reaction*:
   By this point the ground reaction has lost most of its significance as the majority of weight is borne on the other foot.
— *The hip* is in extension and continues to flex as a result of the plantar flexion of the foot and the hip flexors.
— *The knee* is flexed to about 40° and continues to flex under the small ground reaction moment and plantar flexion of the foot.
— *The ankle* has reached 20° of plantar flexion because of contraction of the calf muscles.

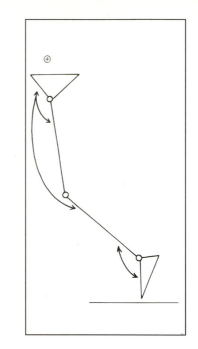

Fig. 8.14 Acceleration. (Reproduced from Hughes J, Jacobs N 1979 Normal human locomotion. Prosthetics and Orthotics International 3: 4–12, by kind permission of the authors and publishers.)

These muscles become inactive directly after toe off.

Acceleration (Fig. 8.14)

— *The hip* is in nearly full extension and flexes as the hip flexors accelerate the limb forward.
— *The knee* is in 40° of flexion and continues to flex to 65° of flexion as a result of contraction of hamstrings and under pendulum action as the limb accelerates.
— *The ankle* is in 20° of plantar flexion directly after toe off. It then begins to actively dorsiflex.

Mid swing (Fig. 8.15)

— *The hip* is flexed to about 20° and continues to flex.
— *The knee* reaches about 65° flexion, then begins to extend under pendulum action and the contraction of the quadriceps muscle.
— *The ankle* has reached neutral and is held there by slight activity of the dorsiflexors.

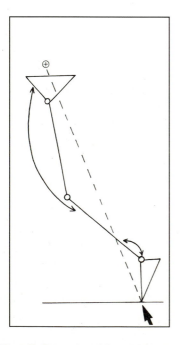

Fig. 8.13 Toe off. (Reproduced from Hughes J, Jacobs N 1979 Normal human locomotion. Prosthetics and Orthotics International 3: 4–12, by kind permission of the authors and publishers.)

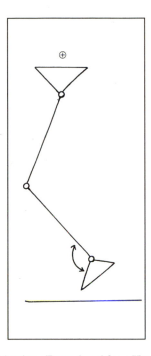

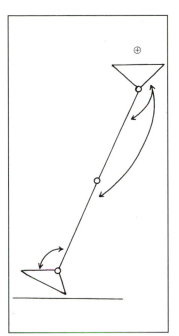

Fig. 8.15 Mid swing. (Reproduced from Hughes J, Jacobs N 1979 Normal human locomotion. Prosthetics and Orthotics International 3: 4–12, by kind permission of the authors and publishers.)

Fig. 8.16 Deceleration. ((Reproduced from Hughes J, Jacobs N 1979 Normal human locomotion. Prosthetics and Orthotics International 3: 4–12, by kind permission of the authors and publishers.)

Deceleration (Fig. 8.16)

— *The hip* reaches 25° of flexion and is restrained by the extensors.
— *The knee* is in extension and is restrained by the hamstrings.
— *The ankle* is held in neutral by the dorsiflexors.

Prosthetic considerations

It is not possible to replace all the movements involved in normal locomotion with prosthetic components. Also, the individual patient is not always capable of managing sophisticated components. The DSC doctor and the prosthetist will try and match the patient's abilities with the components available, and the physiotherapist must retrain the gait, bearing in mind the patient's ability and the design of prosthesis supplied. The diagrams in Tables 8.1 and 8.2 attempt to show the prosthetic components currently available which act during the gait cycle in the sagittal plane.

Analysis in the frontal plane (Fig. 8.17)

Moments in the frontal plane are products of the ground reaction force which passes from a point under the supporting foot through the CG. All moments will be in the direction of adduction at hip and knee and principally inversion at the ankle.

At the hip, the maximal adduction moments occur just before foot flat when maximal vertical load is being applied, and maximal lateral displacement of the pelvis occurs. The patient, therefore, must have strong hip adductor muscles to overcome this adductor moment, otherwise a Trendelenberg gait is produced.

At the knee, the adductor moment is controlled by the integrity of the ligaments, rather than muscular control.

At the ankle the movements of inversion and eversion, which take place mainly at the subtalar joint, control the foot position in this plane.

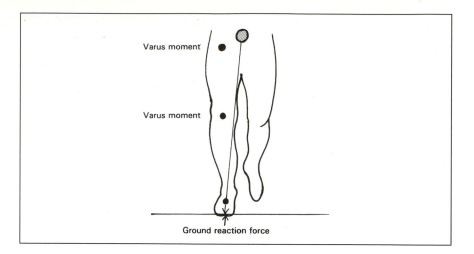

Fig. 8.17   Frontal analysis.

Prosthetic considerations

At the hip, the AK socket design and suspension will assist the control of the adduction moment.

At the foot, the multiaxial ankle and DER feet (see Ch. 7) will help to absorb inversion and eversion, as will the type of shoe worn, e.g. a softer shoe.

Analysis in the transverse plane

A set of complex transverse rotations take place in the pelvis, hip joint, femur and tibia. The swinging limb pivots about its long axis in an outward direction and is suddenly pivoted in the opposite direction at full weightbearing or at the moment of foot flat.

Swing phase is characterised by the external rotation of all segments. The leg segments rotate in the same direction as, and in phase with, pelvic rotation.

Stance phase from heel strike to foot flat is characterised by internal rotation of the segments of the leg.

Prosthetic considerations

The rotation factor is of great importance to the amputee, as in all but the hip disarticulation level the kinetic factors of hip motion are still present. When the amputee walks in a prosthesis, these rotation forces are transmitted down through the prosthesis to the ground, tending to rotate it in the transverse plane. These forces are absorbed at the stump/socket interface where friction can result, and this is a major source of discomfort and skin breakdown. The amputee may then display various gait abnormalities to try and reduce this socket discomfort.

The physiotherapist can try applying a nylon stump sock next to the skin in an attempt to eliminate some of this friction.

Prosthetic components available to absorb some of the rotation forces are torque absorbers and DER feet.

ENERGY COST OF AMBULATION

Much research has been carried out on the amount of energy required by physically fit people when they are walking; this has been compared with the amount of energy required by amputees walking similar distances. The amount of energy required by amputees is significantly greater than that required by normal people, and it varies, depending upon the level of amputation, the reason for amputation, the prosthetic design, the age of the patient and the speed of walking. The average speed of walking for a normally fit person is about 2.5 m.p.h. Any disabled person with gait problems will require more energy to walk the same distance at a similar speed, and amputees, as well as other disabled, tend to walk more slowly than their natural walking speed in order to keep their energy consumption to a minimum. However, the amputee with a higher level of amputation, who has to walk with a stiff knee gait for safety and confidence, will require more energy than a fitter amputee with the same level of amputation who walks with a free knee. Any amputee trying to achieve a normal walking speed over a distance will always use more energy than a normal subject.

Examples of the energy consumption required at different levels of amputation will be found in many research papers, but the findings vary, depending upon the factors measured. However, in general terms, the following applies:

— Unilateral below-knee amputees require up to 9% more mean oxygen consumption than normals

— Unilateral above-knee amputees require up to 49% more mean oxygen consumption than normals

— Bilateral above-knee amputees require up to 280% more mean oxygen consumption than normals (Huang et al 1979).

TECHNIQUES OF GAIT ANALYSIS

To most physiotherapists working in general hospitals and departments, the only method of gait analysis is by clinical observation and the only method of recording is by making notes on the patient's record card.

However, as more specialist university and college departments are becoming interested in gait analysis and its relevance to physiotherapy, our profession is now, is some areas, in contact

Table 8.1 Prosthetic components available during the stance phase

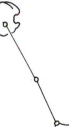

	Heel strike	Foot flat	Mid stance	Heel off	Toe off
Hip joint components	Stride limiter ———————————————————————————————————→				
	Four-bar linkage (geometry) ——————————→				
	Alignment ——→				
Knee joint components	Four-bar linkage (geometry) ——————————→				
	Stance flex ———————————————————————→				
	Extension stop ————→				
	Stabilisers ————————————————————→				
	Swing phase controls (actioned by the movement of flexion) - - - - - - - - - - - - →				
	Alignment ——→				
Foot components	SACH foot rubber density ————————————————————————→				
	Energy-conserving feet ———————————————————————————→				
	Stiffness of rubber components ——————————————————→				
	Heel height adjuster ———————————————————————————→				
	Alignment ——→				

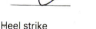

Table 8.2   Prosthetic components available during the swing phase

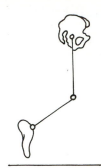 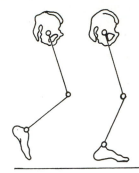 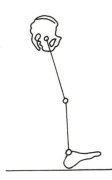

	Acceleration	Mid swing	Deceleration

Acceleration   Mid swing   Deceleration

	Acceleration	Mid swing	Deceleration
Hip joint component	Extension stop Four-bar linkage (geometry) ———— Position of the hip joint (geometry) ————————		Flexion stop ——————————▶ ——————————▶
		Stride limiter ———————	——————▶
	Alignment ————————		——————————▶

Knee joint components	Swing phase controls,
	  e.g. pneumatic,
	  hydraulic, other ———
	  mechanical devises
	Alignment ————————
			——————————▶
			
			——————————▶

Foot components	_____	_____	_____

Table 8.3   Techniques of gait analysis (reproduced by kind permission of Dr M Whittle)

Technique	Diagnosis	Usefulness of information			Expense
		Assessment	Monitoring	Research	
1 *Visual gait analysis* (movements only) The principal factor here is the skill and experience of the clinician. No objective data are collected	★	★			None
2. *Videotape analysis* The patient can observe their own gait. The clinicians may observe the gait repeatedly, to do a more detailed analysis, including in slow motion. The tape can be kept as a record	★	★	★	★	Moderate
3. *Velocity, cadence* A stopwatch and pocket calculator are required Velocity = time over a known distance Cadence = no. of footfalls in a given time		★	★★	★	Cheap

Table 8.3   (cont'd)

Technique	Diagnosis	Usefulness of information			Expense
		Assessment	Monitoring	Research	
4. *Foot placement* The patient steps in talcum powder then walks across the floor. Step and stride lengths, width of walking base and foot contact pattern can be examined and measured		★	★★	★	Cheap (but messy)
5. *Foot pressure distribution* Information concerning foot pressure and its relation to the centre of gravity can be gained by pedobarograph and other devices. Some systems have the capacity for dynamic examination, and some measure pressure within the shoe	★★	★★	★	★★★	Expensive
6. *Gait timing* This uses foot switches or an instrumented walkway. It measures cadence, stance and swing phase times and single and double support times		★	★★	★	Expensive
7. *Electrogoniometry* Measurement of joint movement in one or more planes. It is cumbersome and requires strapping to the leg which in itself may alter the natural gait pattern. Electrogoniometers and others are used		★	★★	★★	Moderate
8. *Force platforms* These measure the force applied by the foot to the ground. Simple models record only vertical force and centre of pressure; more expensive ones record horizontal and vertical forces		★	★★	★★	Expensive
9. *Electromyography* This records the action potentials of muscle working at any point in the gait cycle. Electrodes may be placed on the skin over a muscle or fine wires are inserted into it. This gives little information about muscle forces. It is mainly of use with neurological or myopathic disorders	★★	★★★	★★	★★	Expensive
		(in specific conditions only)			
10. *Kinematics* This entails the use of cine or television cameras, possibly linked to a computer, to measure limb movement in 2 or 3 dimensions	★	★★	★★	★★	Very expensive
11. *Combined kinetic/kinematic system* This involves the use of a forceplatform with a kinematic system and can also be used with an EMG. It measures joint moments and angles and force transmission	★	★★★	★★★	★★★	Very expensive
12. *Heart rare measurement* Gives an indirect indication of the energy being expended in walking	★	★	★	★	Cheap
13. *Oxygen uptake* Gives an almost direct measurement of the energy being expended in walking	★	★★	★★	★★	Expensive

Assessment refers to a single examination.
Monitoring refers to a series of examinations over a period of time.

with clinical physiologists and bio-engineers who have more specialist equipment available for our use. Table 8.3 lists some techniques which the physiotherapists may encounter.

ACKNOWLEDGEMENTS

The authors acknowledge teaching material from the University of Strathclyde, Glasgow, New York University, and Northwestern University, Chicago, USA.

REFERENCES

Bard G, Ralston H J 1959 Measurement of energy expenditure during ambulation with special reference to the evaluation of assistive devices. Archives of Physical Medicine and Rehabilitation 40: 415–420

Fisher S V 1978 Energy cost of ambulation in health and disability. A literature review. Archives of Physical Medicine and Rehabilitation 59: 124–133

Gailey R, Kirk N 1991 Energy expenditure of below-knee amputees during unrestrained ambulation. WCPT 11th International Congress Proceedings Book II: 650–652

Ganguli S, Datta S R, Chatterjee B B, Roy B N 1974 Metabolic cost of walking at different speeds with patellar tendon-bearing prosthesis. Journal of Applied Physiology 36(4): 440–443

Huang C T, Jackson J R, Moore N B et al 1979 Amputation: energy cost of ambulation. Archives of Physical Medicine and Rehabilitation 60: 18–24

Hughes J, Jacobs N 1979 Normal human locomotion. Prosthetics and Orthotics International 3: 4–12

Little H 1981 Gait analysis for physiotherapy departments: a review of current methods. Physiotherapy 67(11): 334–337

Netz, Weisen, Wetterberg 1981 Videotape recording — a complementary aid for the walking training of lower limb amputees. Prosthetics and Orthotics International 5: 147–150

Nowroozi F, Salvenelli M 1983 Energy expenditure in hip disarticulation and hemipelvectomy amputees. Archives of Physical Medicine and Rehabilitation 64(7): 300–303

Patla A E, Proctor J, Morson B 1987 Observations on aspects of visual gait assessment: a questionnaire study. Physiotherapy Canada 39(5): 311–316

Robinson J L, Smidt G L 1981 Quantitative gait evaluation in the clinic. Physical Therapy 61(3): 351–353

Rose G K 1983 Clinical gait assessment: a personal view. Journal of Medical Engineering and Technology 7(6): 273–279

Saunders J B de C N, Inman V T, Eberhart H D 1953 The major determinant in normal and pathological gait. Journal of Bone and Joint Surgery 35–A: 543–548

Sethi P K 1977 The foot and footwear. Prosthetics and Orthotics International 1(3): 173–182

Smith D M, Lord M, Kinnear E M L 1983 A video aid to assessment and retraining of standing balance. In: Perkins W J (ed) High technology aids for the disabled. Butterworths, London

Winter D A 1980 Overall principle of lower limb support during stance phase of gait. Journal of Biomechanics 13: 923–927

9. Gait re-education

Ideally, prosthetic rehabilitation should take place as part of in-patient care, as a more successful functional outcome is achieved and the patient is discharged with a 'complete' body image. However, many hospitals have constraints on their beds and prosthetic rehabilitation takes place on an out-patient basis.

As the patient will have been mobile using an early walking aid, e.g. Ppam aid, and will have had gait re-education within the limits of the device, it is important there is continuity from this stage to the prosthetic stage. If there is a delay in organising an appointment the amputee may attempt to use the prosthesis, and as a result will usually produce a poor walking pattern which is difficult to alter later on, even with expert tuition. Some older amputees will sit and await instruction; delay will result in their physical condition deteriorating and the prostheses will no longer fit them. Therefore, the hospital physiotherapist must keep in contact with patients, whether they are still in hospital or at home and be aware of all prosthetic appointments and delivery dates.

Planning of transport arrangements to the physiotherapy department must be made. Not all physiotherapy departments are able to arrange gait re-education (this is usually because of transport difficulties) so that referral to another hospital, day hospital or physiotherapy department must be made. These arrangements are time-consuming and difficult but must be pursued with vigour. If none of these arrangements is possible then referral to the community physiotherapist is made. Indeed, the home environment can be the most relevant place for retraining functional activity.

Treatment should be on a daily basis, but it may be necessary to fit the physiotherapy around visits from home helps and district nurses, and clinic appointments. The patients should attend for a whole morning or afternoon, or both, so that sufficient time is given to exercise, walking and rest periods. Treatment does not have to be on a one-to-one basis; a rehabilitation environment is preferable, e.g. in a gymnasium where several patients can be treated simultaneously.

The advantages of daily treatment are:

1. Continuity of treatment improves prosthetic re-education and acceptance of the prosthesis by the patient.

2. The patient adjusts more quickly to the new body image.

3. The skin toughens more quickly to tolerate new weightbearing areas.

4. Functional activities other than walking are practised, e.g. putting on and taking off the prosthesis, attending meals and sitting in different chairs, using the lavatory and walking outside the actual treatment area. All activities must be relevant to the amputee's individual needs.

5. Independence using the prosthesis is achieved more quickly. For example, a single below-knee amputee may only need 1 week of gait re-education; the single above-knee amputee may only need 2 weeks of gait re-education, but the bilateral amputee, particularly without natural knee joints, is more likely to take over a month to walk with reasonable independence.

PATIENT CONSIDERATIONS

The pattern of walking exhibited by an individual represents his solution to the problem of how to get from one place to another with minimum effort, adequate stability and acceptable appearance. The relative importance attached to each of these aspects differs from one individual to another.

As stated in Chapter 8, the appearance of normal gait is the sum total of the various characteristic determinants of human locomotion. The gait of an amputee will depend upon the condition of the determinants remaining, e.g. joints, skeletal links, muscles, body shape and weight, the extent to which the prosthetic replacements mimic the original body parts and the interface between body and prosthesis.

Before starting gait re-education it is important that the physiotherapist has realistic goals in mind and discusses these with the patient. The following points should be considered while assessing the patient at the first treatment session (see Chs 2 and 6):

— Diagnosis
— Other medical problems
— Life expectancy
— Age
— Physical state and functional capabilities
— State of psychological adjustment
— Social and housing situation
— The patient's expectations with the prosthesis supplied.

Initial stages

The physiotherapist must follow an organised sequence of re-examination of the patient and detailed inspection of the prosthesis even before applying the prosthesis.

Examination of the patient

All the features of the original examination database (see Ch. 2) are re-checked or, if the patient is new to the physiotherapist, carried out in full. Particular emphasis is now paid to the mobility of the trunk which plays such a large part in the maintenance of a symmetrical gait pattern.

Inspection of the stump

In addition to the general examination of range of movement and muscle power, the stump should be inspected for shape, muscle cover, distal bone bevelling, areas of skin redness or breakdown and a close inspection is made of the scar. If the scar is unhealed, or adherent to the underlying soft tissue or bone, it will suffer trauma when in the close fitting socket of the prosthesis and therefore the length of time that the prosthesis is worn must be limited. This is particularly important with the below-knee level in a patellar tendon bearing prosthesis (see Ch. 13).

Check of the prosthesis

The prosthesis is checked on its own, BEFORE the patient applies it. Unless all the features of the prosthesis are understood by the therapist, correct gait training will be impossible. A careful inspection must be made of the:

— *suspension, joints and socket* (see relevant level chapter for details)
— *static alignment and shoe.* A prosthesis should stand on its own on a flat surface without any support. If the shoe is not the one for which the limb was made, the prosthesis will appear to incline either forwards or backwards, as the keel of the prosthetic foot will not be correctly balanced by the heel height of the shoe.

The stump sock

There are many different types of sock (see Ch. 7) and the first prosthesis for a primary amputee should ideally fit with one wool sock, but as stump volume varies considerably in the early stages, a variety of socks should have been supplied. The physiotherapist can then experiment with them in order to achieve the correct fit of the socket (see the relevant level chapters).

Check of the fit of the prosthesis

The weightbearing areas, suspension, length, alignment and comfort must all be checked prior to gait re-education (see relevant level chapters for detail).

In the parallel bars

All gait re-education should start in the parallel bars. However, if these are not available, e. g. in a patient's home, a suitably safe support should be devised, such as holding a fixed work surface or chair back.

With the feet at a normal base width (i.e. 5–10 cms) and with both hands holding the bars, weight transference is attempted over the prosthesis. The aim is for the supporting limb to be in the mid-line of the body. This can be assisted by the physiotherapist directing the movement of the pelvis and shoulder manually and progressing to a resisted movement. This side-to-side weight transference is then practised with the contralateral hand only holding the bar and progressed to the ipsilateral hand only, which is harder. Rhythmic stabilisations in standing with a normal base width, and then stride standing are practised to encourage balance.

After these preliminary exercises, and frequent rests if required, walking is then started holding both bars, and stepping off with the sound limb. The aim is for a symmetrical gait pattern; this is achieved when the pelvis moves forward over the supporting limb, equal stride length is made, correct reciprocal trunk movements occur and the hands are advanced in the correct rhythm. The physiotherapist must be inside the parallel bars, giving guidance to the pelvis, shoulder or prosthesis and either assisting the movement or resisting it.

Many patients find achievement of a symmetrical gait pattern difficult, and unless sufficient time and manual guidance are given at this early stage, gait faults appear. Walking must continue in the bars in a forward, sideways and backwards direction, paying particular attention to reciprocal trunk rotation.

Progression out of the parallel bars

Progression from here is dependent on the general capabilities of the individual patient. Most primary amputees of all levels should aim to walk with two sticks, progressing to one when the skin of weightbearing areas has more tolerance and strength, balance and confidence have improved. If crutches are used, none of the progression described above occurs and progression in amputee gait training is inhibited. The walking frame is the last resort for the amputee, as it forces the hips into flexion, causing incorrect weightbearing areas on the socket; the pelvis does not move vertically over the supporting limb, the trunk cannot rotate and a symmetrical pattern is impossible.

The gait pattern that is adopted in the early stages of rehabilitation becomes fixed in the amputee's mind; therefore it is worth all the time and resource implications in these early sessions to aim for a good gait pattern with walking sticks. Retraining the patient with sticks after they have used crutches or a frame is extremely difficult and often unsuccessful.

The young fit unilateral amputee

The aim of re-education for this amputee is always to attain a normal gait pattern. Full strength of all muscle groups and full mobility of trunk and all joints are essential to achieve this. The exercise programme should be concurrent with prosthetic education.

Observation of the patient can only be carried out if the patient is suitably undressed in order that arms, trunk, spine, hips and knees are clearly visible. Observation of the whole body should be made, from head to foot, from the front, the sides and from behind.

The patient then progresses to using two sticks; these aids are necessary to prevent any gait deviation as a result of skin soreness from the weightbearing areas. Sticks should not be discarded too quickly as deterioration of the gait pattern can occur.

Visual feedback of performance can be aided by the use of mirrors or video equipment to reinforce the physiotherapist's instructions.

The rehabilitation programme must be fitted around other important aspects of the patient's life, e.g. school, college or employment. The importance of follow-up visits is discussed so that checks on the gait pattern are maintained; the young amputee can easily adopt an incorrect gait pattern during the early stages of prosthetic use. Also, progression of mobility into leisure activities at sports can be advised at the right time (see Ch. 15).

There is, however, a group of patients whose gait pattern deteriorates after discharge from physiotherapy. This is thought to be because of a psychological need to present to others a visible disability. These patients are often quite capable of walking normally but choose not to do so. The physiotherapist must be aware of this so that at follow-up visits the emphasis is on psychological support rather than criticism of the observed gait. This may gradually improve as the patient adjusts to the new situation.

The older unilateral amputee

The aim for this amputee is to attain the best possible gait pattern, bearing in mind that certain physical problems (e.g. flexion contracture, claudication, cardiorespiratory limitation) may limit normal pattern. A daily exercise programme will minimise their effects.

First, a check is made to see if the patient can put on and take off the prosthesis, and advice is given if there are clothing difficulties. After initial instruction from the physiotherapist, patients can be left to practise on their own for short periods when it is safe to do so; rest periods should be allowed as much as required. Further instruction and correction are given as necessary. The use of mirrors at this stage helps some patients, giving visual feedback of the gait pattern.

For these patients progress is slow but steady. It has been found that daily attendance for gait re-education hastens mobility and the use of just one, or two, sticks can be achieved. Social activities and activities of daily living should then be encouraged. Consideration of home environment and confidence levels are as important as physical ability.

Following discharge, review and treatment are necessary when the prescription of the prosthesis changes, or if the medical condition alters.

The frail elderly amputee and those with multiple medical problems

The rehabilitation aims for these amputees are safety and function. The actual gait pattern achieved is irrelevant and formal gait training unnecessary. The most important task is to identify the individual patient's needs by visiting the home environment.

In the physiotherapy department the patient first learns how to put on and take off the prosthesis. This process may take some time to achieve and adaptations to the suspension of the prosthesis may be helpful. There is little point in continuing with the prosthesis if the patient cannot apply it independently when no help is available at home.

The patient must not only learn to walk, but must be able to stand up from and sit down on a chair without overbalancing. Transfers must be performed safely; these patients cannot afford to fall as the result may prove to be catastrophic.

Short treatment sessions spaced throughout the day, with simple but repetitive activity, have been found to achieve the best result. This group needs to be treated symptomatically; if they are unwell for the occasional session they should be allowed to rest. However, a little activity should be tried each day.

The physiotherapist must be aware that this group of patients may not succeed in using a prosthesis. If there is no indication that independence will be achieved, even after a fair trial, then a positive decision must be made with the patient and carer to stop gait re-education. A wheelchair must then be used and the patient fully instructed and assessed in its use.

For those who are progressing, the walking aid chosen must be the safest in the home surroundings: for many this will be a walking frame.

Once a comfortable fit of the prosthesis has been achieved, and the patient is safe while walking, the community physiotherapist should be contacted. Functional activities within the home can continue and other members of the primary health care team can give support. Treatment in the physiotherapy department then ceases but may be restarted, for a short intensive period, if referral back from the community is made. An example of this is if the patient stops using the prosthesis because of a short illness, e.g. chest infection, abdominal operation or immobility following a fall, etc.

Those patients with progressive disease and the frail elderly may find that prostheses are of no functional use and in no way enhance the quality of their life. Careful assessment and exploration of their thoughts and feelings should be sensitively made before returning the prosthesis to the DSC. Some patients feel that their prosthesis, which they have had for some time, is a real part of them and suffer a reaction if it is removed against their wishes.

The bilateral amputee

The aim of gait re-education is governed by:

— The presence of natural knee joints
— The ability to apply the prostheses
— Associated diseases
— Adequate cardiorespiratory status
— Home environment (see Chs 6 and 16).

The bilateral below-knee amputee will achieve a normal gait pattern but other levels will almost always appear unnatural. The gait pattern achieved and successful prosthetic outcome will depend on the levels of amputation.

In the physiotherapy department, the patient is taught how to put on and take off the prostheses. This requires time, patience, perseverance and much practice. The patient then dresses and commences walking in the parallel bars. Standing up and sitting down can be difficult and requires considerable practice and experimentation using different chair designs. The patient remains in the parallel bars for many treatment sessions, as balance takes some time to achieve and skin tolerance takes time to build up.

The energy required to use two prostheses is very high and time should be allowed for patients to gradually increase their stamina: the higher the levels of amputation, the greater the energy cost when walking.

Once some balance has been achieved, the patient progresses to using walking aids: the choice is between quadrapods and walking sticks. It is not safe for a bilateral amputee to use a frame as the base is not always wide enough for the patient's stance; there is a tendency for the bilateral amputee to fall backwards whilst lifting the frame and the considerable side-to-side trunk sway required to initiate swing phase may make the frame tip sideways. The advantages of quadrapods are that they are stable, free standing and can be correctly positioned before the patient stands up. The disadvantage is that the combined

width of patient and quadrapods is considerable; this is a point to consider if the patient lives in a small home.

If, after a fair trial of gait re-education throughout several sessions, the patient is unable to walk outside the parallel bars using aids, then it is obvious that prosthetic use will not enhance the patient's lifestyle. A positive decision must be made with the patient to stop using prostheses, to continue rehabilitation in a suitable wheelchair and explore leisure activities.

For those patients who are able to walk with aids, the physiotherapist must visit their homes to see if they can manage. It may be apparent that even though the patient can walk well in the physiotherapy department, prosthetic use at home may be a hindrance.

For those who manage well, follow-up treatment sessions will be necessary when the prosthetic prescription changes.

Bilateral amputees require a great deal of time (2–3 hours) for each treatment session. Nothing can be achieved in a typical half-hour out-patient session and the physiotherapist must take this into account when organising the place and time of treatment. The exercise programme should continue concurrently with prosthetic education.

GAIT ANALYSIS

The gait should first be analysed visually in the parallel bars. An overall view of the whole patient is taken from the front, at the side and from behind. It is often helpful if the physiotherapist sits on a low stool to observe movement of the pelvis and legs. The analysis then proceeds to observing the gait pattern during both stance and swing phases. This analysis is carried out at every treatment session. A table of detailed gait analysis techniques is given in Chapter 8. Common gait faults are given in Tables 9.1 and 9.2.

Any observed deviation should be noted. It is important that these deviations are expressed in standard terminology used by a prosthetist, so that discussion between the hospital physiotherapist and the prosthetist is readily understandable.

Table 9.1   Gait analysis of the below-knee level using a patellar tendon bearing prosthesis

Deviation	Amputee cause	Prosthetic cause
1. *Excessive knee flexion* during stance phase	1. Fixed flexion of knee and hip joint 2. Habit 3. Pain	1. Excessive dorsiflexion of prosthetic foot 2. Socket incorrectly aligned: either insufficient flexion set in the socket, or the whole shin set too far forward on the foot 3. Socket ill-fitting 4. Cuff suspension faulty 5. Excessively stiff plantar flexion of prosthetic foot
2. *Insufficient knee flexion or hyperextension* during the stance phase N.B. PTB sockets are aligned with 15° flexion	1. Weakness of vastus medialis muscle 2. Knee joint instability 3. Stump discomfort 4. Particularly common if amputee is used to a thigh corset prosthesis as the patient has difficulty establishing this new knee pattern	1. Excessive plantar flexion of foot 2. Too hard a plantar flexion resistance 3. Socket incorrectly aligned: either too flexed or shin set too far back on the foot
3. *Rotation of foot*	1. Weak muscles around the hip 2. Knee joint instability combined with knee muscle weakness 3. Pain	1. Too hard a plantar flexion resistance 2. Ill-fitting socket 3. Poor suspension
4. *Lateral shift of the prosthesis* during stance phase	1. Stump pain	1. Incorrect alignment of prosthesis: socket too abducted or the foot is set too far medially
5. *Lateral bending of the trunk* during stance phase (patient leans towards the prosthesis)	1. Painful stump or pain in the remaining leg 2. Lack of balance 3. Lack of confidence 4. Muscle imbalance, weakness at the hip joint	1. Prosthesis too short 2. Incorrect alignment: socket too adducted or the foot is set too far laterally
6. *Drop off* Knee flexion occurs too early in stance phase	1. No identifiable cause	1. Excessive dorsiflexion of foot 2. Incorrect alignment: socket set too far forward
7. *Delayed knee flexion* during the swing phase	1. Problems with pelvic and hip movements 2. Knee joint stiffness 3. Habit, after having used an AK/BK prosthesis	1. Inadequate suspension
8. *General deviations*	1. Uneven arm swing 2. Uneven timing 3. Uneven steps 4. Patient too tired to maintain a good gait pattern	

AK/BK, above-knee/below-knee

Table 9.2 Gait analysis of the above-knee and through-knee levels of amputation. Each individual patient can only be expected to walk within their capabilities. Some gait deviations may occur because the prosthesis is too complicated for the individual. After a fair trial of gait re-education, the physiotherapist should contact the prosthetist if there are problems, and suggest either modifications or a change of prescription

Deviation	Stiff knee gait		Free knee gait	
	Amputee causes	Prosthetic causes	Amputee causes	Prosthetic causes
1. *Abducted pattern* Patient walking with wide base with prosthesis held away from the mid line	1. Abduction contracture of stump 2. Adductor roll 3. Habit pattern	1. Prosthesis too long 2. Medial brim of socket too high therefore causing discomfort on the pubic ramus 3. Lateral wall of socket giving insufficient support to femur 4. Rigid pelvic band incorrect 5. Prosthesis incorrectly aligned: socket too adducted	Same reasons	Same reasons
2. *Lateral or side bending of the trunk* during stance phase	*Towards prosthetic side* 1. Abduction contracture of stump 2. Very short stump 3. Painful or sensitive stump 4. Habit pattern	1. Lateral wall of the socket may give insufficient support to the femur 2. Prosthesis too short 3. Prosthesis incorrectly aligned: socket too adducted 4. Medial brim of the socket giving discomfort causing pattern to lean away from it	Same reasons	Same reasons
	Away from prosthetic side 1. Weak abductors on stump side	1. Prosthesis too long 2. Prosthesis incorrectly aligned: socket too abducted	Same reasons	Same reasons
3. *Rotation of foot at heel strike* usually outwards	1. Poor muscle control of the stump, extensors and medial rotators	1. Plantar flexion resistance too hard 2. Socket may be too loose 3. Prosthesis incorrectly aligned (too much toe out)	Same reasons	Same reasons

Table 9.2 (cont'd)

Deviation	Stiff knee gait		Free knee gait	
	Amputee causes	Prosthetic causes	Amputee causes	Prosthetic causes
4. *Circumduction* Prosthesis is swung in a wide arc during swing phase	1. Abduction contracture of stump 2. Muscle imbalance: weak adductors of the stump and inability to hip hitch 3. Habit pattern	1. Prosthesis too long 2. Inadequate suspension	1. Same reasons 2. Muscle weakness 3. Lack of confidence in flexing the knee	1. Same reasons 2. Too much stability, or too much friction in the knee mechanism
5. *Vaulting* The patient rises up on the toe of the remaining leg to swing the prosthesis through from toe off to heel strike	1. Fear of catching the toe of the prosthesis 2. Very short stump 3. Poor muscle control (hip hitching) 4. Habit pattern	1. Prosthesis too long 2. Inadequate suspension	1. Same reasons 2. Poor muscle control of hip flexion	1. Same reasons 2. Too much stability or friction in the knee mechanism
6. *Uneven step length*	*Prosthetic too long* (most common) 1. Inability to extend hip over prosthesis during stance phase, due to hip flexion contracture and weakness of hip and back extensors 2. Lack of confidence 3. Habit pattern, especially if initial gait rehabilitation was using a frame for aid *Short prosthetic step* 1. Lack of confidence 2. Pain	1. Flexion contracture not accommodated prosthetically 2. Prosthesis too long 1. Ill-fitting socket causing discomfort 2. Alignment incorrect: socket too flexed	*Prosthetic step too long* 1. Same reasons 2. Habit, to ensure prosthesis is flung into extension *Short prosthetic step* (most common) 1. Patient feels insecure with the free knee mechanism	1. Same reasons 1. Prosthetic knee may buckle because of incorrect alignment or adjustment: socket too flexed
7. *Uneven timing* Steps of unequal length usually characterised by a very short stance phase on the prosthesis	1. Lack of balance 2. Lack of confidence 3. Weak stump, trunk and remaining leg muscles 4. Habit pattern 5. Pain on the ischial seating	1. Ill-fitting socket causing discomfort	Same reasons in free knee gait as 6	Same reasons in free knee gait as 6

Table 9.2 (cont'd)

Deviation	Stiff knee gait		Free knee gait	
	Amputee causes	Prosthetic causes	Amputee causes	Prosthetic causes
8. *Uneven arm swing* The arm on the prosthetic side is usually held stiff to that side of the body. There is no natural swing	1. Lack of balance 2. Lack of confidence 3. Habit pattern	1. Ill-fitting socket causing discomfort	Same reasons in free knee gait as 6 & 7	Same reasons in free knee gait as 6 & 7
	N.B. Uneven step length, uneven timing and uneven arm swing are often seen in combination and are often a result of the same cause			
9. *Lumbar lordosis* During stance phase there is excessive curvature of the lumbar spine	1. Hip flexion contracture 2. Weak hip extensors 3. Weak abdominal muscles 4. Attempt to move centre of gravity forwards to improve stability 5. Habit pattern	1. Insufficient flexion in socket alignment 2. Discomfort on ischial weightbearing area 3. Heel of shoe on prosthesis too high	Same reasons	1. Same reasons 2. Insufficient stability in knee mechanism
10. *Forward trunk flexion*	1. Weak hip extensors 2. Hip flexion contracture 3. Poor general posture 4. Kyphosed spine 5. Habit pattern looking at feet, from walking with a frame, or because of poor eyesight	1. Insufficient flexion built into socket 2. Socket discomfort	Same reasons	1. Same reasons 2. Insufficient knee stability in mechanism
11. *Drop off* There is a downwards movement of the body as weight is transferred forwards over the prosthetic foot	1. Wearing the incorrect shoe	1. Too soft a dorsiflexion resistance in prosthetic foot 2. Socket too anterior to the foot	Same reasons	Same reasons
12. *Foot slap* Prosthetic forefoot audibly slaps down onto floor at heel strike	1. Habit pattern of driving prosthetic heel into ground excessively 2. Wearing incorrect shoe for the set of prosthetic foot	1. Plantar flexion resistance too soft. It does not offer sufficient resistance as weight is transferred onto the prosthesis	Same reasons	Same reasons

Table 9.2 (cont'd)

Deviation	Stiff knee gait		Free knee gait	
	Amputee causes	Prosthetic causes	Amputee causes	Prosthetic causes
13. *Uneven heel rise* Heel of prosthesis rises upwards excessively when knee flexes at beginning of swing phase	N/A	N/A	1. Too much hip flexor muscle power used to flex the prosthetic knee	1. Prosthetic knee flexes too easily 2. Swing phase controls adjusted incorrectly
14. a. *Medial whip* Heel travels medially on initial flexion at beginning of swing phase	N/A	N/A	*Medial* Walking habits caused by stump discomfort or a problem in the remaining leg	*Medial* Excessive external rotation of prosthetic knee *Lateral* Excessive internal rotation of prosthetic knee *Generally* 1. The socket may be too tight a fit 2. The socket may be too loose 3. Incorrect alignment at toe off 4. Excessive valgus or varus set into the prosthesis at the knee level
b. *Lateral whip* Heel travels laterally on initial flexion at beginning of swing phase	N/A	N/A	*Lateral* Same as above	
15. *Terminal swing impact* Knee reaches extension too quickly prior to heel strike	N/A	N/A	1. Stump forcibly flexes to produce full extension of the knee to ensure safety 2. Habit 3. Lack of confidence This is often seen in combination with too long a prosthetic step	1. Incorrect adjustment of swing phase controls

Causes of gait deviation

These may be:

1. The general condition of the patient
2. The shape, length and size of the stump and any discomfort present
3. Prosthetic malfunction
4. Inadequate or incorrect re-education
5. Psychological, social or economic reasons.

The purpose of identifying gait deviation and its cause is to improve the gait pattern towards the normal. This may be achieved by medical or surgical treatment, physiotherapeutic measures, psychological help, prosthetic alteration, or by gait re-education. These treatments are to the patient's advantage because the nearer to normal the gait pattern becomes, the less energy is consumed. Therefore, the exercise tolerance is extended, and as a result the patient feels less disabled. However, the physiotherapist often treats the patient during the early stages in which the stump is still maturing and it will be found that many gait deviations will be caused simply by stump discomfort and volumetric changes.

Habit

Each patient's gait is individual and has its own habit pattern. This may have been present before the amputation, but it may have been caused by walking in an uncomfortable prosthesis at an earlier stage without adequate rehabilitation. The former habit pattern cannot usually be evaluated but the latter should have been avoided. Exceptionally, some patients have never been referred for gait re-education and will have taught themselves and managed the best they can.

ACKNOWLEDGEMENTS

The authors acknowledge teaching material form the University of Strathclyde, Glasgow, New York University and Northwestern University, Chicago, USA.

REFERENCES

Breakey J 1976 Gait of unilateral below-knee amputees. Orthotics and Prosthetics 30(3): 17–24

Buttenshaw P Dolman J 1992 The Roehampton approach to rehabilitation: a retrospective survey of prosthetic use in patients with primary unilateral lower limb amputation. Topics in Geriatric Medicine 8(1): 72–78

Culham E G, Peat M, Newell E 1984 Analysis of gait following below-knee amputation: a comparison of the SACH and single-axis foot. Physiotherapy Canada 36 (5): 237–242

Day H J B 1981 The assessment and description of amputee activity. Prosthetics and Orthotics International 5:23–28

Foort J 1979 Alignment of the above-knee prosthesis. Prosthetics and Orthotics International 3: 137–139

Friberg O 1984 Biomechanical significance of the correct length of lower limb prostheses: a clinical and radiological study. Prosthetics and Orthotics International 8: 124–129

Ishai G, Bar A, Susak Z 1983 Effects of alignment variables on thigh axial torque during swing phase in AK amputee gait. Prosthetics and Orthotics International 7: 41–47

Kay J 1991 Domiciliary rehabilitation of elderly amputees. Physiotherapy 77(1): 60–61

Klenerman L, Dobbs R J, Weller C et al 1988 Bringing gait analysis out of the laboratory and into the clinic. Age and Ageing 17: 397–450

Lord M, Smith D M 1984 Foot loading in amputee stance. Prosthetics and Orthotics International 8: 159–164

May D R W, Davis B 1974 Gait and the lower-limb amputee. Physiotherapy 60(6): 166–171

Murray M P et al 1983 Gait patterns in above-knee amputee patients: hydraulic swing control vs constant-friction knee components. Archives of Physical Medicine and Rehabilitation 64: 339–345

Patrick J H 1991 Movement analysis improves diagnostic ability. Medical Audit News I(6): 91–92

Stillman B 1991 Computer-based video analysis of movement. Australian Journal of Physiotherapy 37: 219–227

Saleh M, Murdoch G 1985 In defence of gait analysis: observation and measurement in gait analysis. Journal of Bone and Joint Surgery 67B(2): 237–241

Stillman B 1991 Computer-based video analysis of movement. Australian Journal of Physiotherapy 37: 219–227

Wall J C, Charteris J, Turnbull G I 1987 Two steps equals one stride equals what?: the applicability of normal gait nomenclature to abnormal walking patterns. Clinical Biomechanics 2: 119–125

10. The hemipelvectomy and hip disarticulation levels of amputation

The majority of hemipelvectomy and hip disarticulation levels of amputation are performed for malignant bone tumours in the lower limb. Occasionally, severe vascular disease, osteomyelitis and very rarely severe trauma may also result in the selection of this level of amputation. In exceptional cases it has been known for bilateral hip disarticulation to be caused by trauma.

These are extensive amputations involving the large muscle groups around the pelvis. There is no stump to act as a lever for prosthetic control and mobility is slow. In some cases such extensive surgery may result in slow wound healing and the need for secondary skin grafting. Those who are undergoing chemotherapy and radiotherapy may also have wound healing problems and these patients often feel unwell.

These are very mutilating procedures and many patients find psychological adjustment difficult. All those suffering from malignancy require an enormous amount of psychological help at all stages of their care. Parents may require even more help and support (see Ch. 2).

Hemipelvectomy

Generally, half the pelvis is removed, as well as the total lower limb. It is important to have X-ray confirmation of the extent of bony removal.

Hip disarticulation

This is a true disarticulation of the femur from the acetabulum; the total lower limb is removed, leaving the whole pelvis intact. Some surgeons leave the head of the femur in situ; this can cause great difficulty with socket fitting. This is not a true hip disarticulation but prosthetically is treated as one.

PROSTHESES

As soon as the patient's wound is healed, assessment can be made by the prosthetic rehabilitation team. Provided the patient is sufficiently fit, the prosthetist will take a plaster-of-Paris cast embracing the site of amputation. It is essential that the patient is able to stand for a period of time necessary for this procedure, at least half an hour. Figures 10.1 and 10.2 illustrate lightweight prostheses supplied for this level of amputation.

Socket

The shape of the socket depends always upon the plaster cast of the patient's pelvis. Patients usually have a totally embracing socket, enclosing both iliac crests, made of thermoplastic material. For the hemipelvectomy patient, this contains and supports the abdominal and pelvic contents.

The weightbearing areas of the socket are different for each level of amputation:
— *Hemipelvectomy*: the patient's weight has to be transferred over to the ischial tuberosity and buttock of the remaining leg
— *Hip disarticulation*: the patient's weight is taken through the ischium and buttock of the amputated side.

Suspension

The suspension of these sockets is achieved through the total tissue contact, locking over the iliac crests; occasionally, extra suspension may be supplied by adding a shoulder strap.

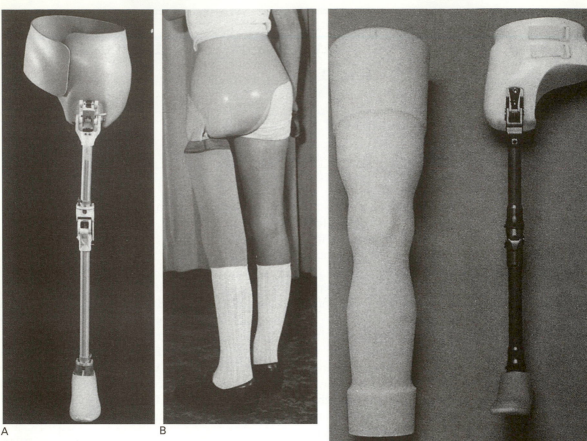

A   B

Fig. 10.1 An Ultra Roelite prosthesis for hip disarticulation. (A) A tilting table hip mechanism and four-bar linkage knee mechanism. (B) The same prosthesis when completed.

Fig. 10.2 Modular hip disarticulation prosthesis for children. (Photograph by kind permission of Otto Bock Orthopaedic (UK) Ltd.)

Hip components

Canadian joint with hip limiter

The mechanism is placed anteriorly on the socket. It allows movement at the hip during the swing phase. Movement is controlled by a limiter, which can be adjusted by the prosthetist to increase or decrease the stride length of the artificial limb. This component can be supplied either with or without a locking mechanism.

Four-bar linkage

The geometric design of this joint gives the advantage of the instantaneous centre of rotation occurring at the natural hip joint level. It therefore gives a smooth and easy gait pattern as it shortens the length of prosthesis during the swing phase,

thus ensuring safe foot clearance of the floor. The component is on the anterior aspect of the socket and fits right out of the way when sitting, making it the most comfortable design (see Fig. 10.3).

Knee components

For a fuller explanation of these mechanisms see Chapter 11.

The popular choice, particularly for new amputees, is the stabilised knee with optional locking mechanism. It allows total stability in up to 22° flexion during stance phase, but otherwise is a free knee. The amputee can choose to lock it totally when the occasion demands.

Another component used is the four-bar linkage, which can also be supplied with a lock.

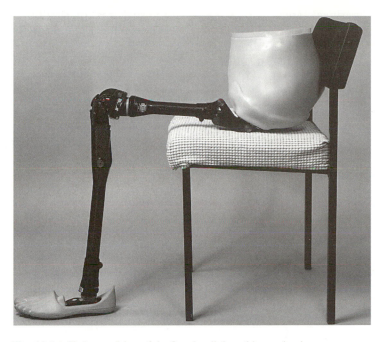

Fig. 10.3   Sitting position of the four-bar linkage hip mechanism. (Photograph by kind permission of C. A. Blatchford & Sons Ltd.)

Prostheses supplied for the hemipelvectomy and hip disarticulation levels of amputation may have any combination of the hip and knee joints described above. It is important that the physiotherapist understands the various components and looks at them in detail, in order that the patient can be instructed correctly.

CHECK OF THE PROSTHESIS

The fit of the prosthesis must be checked by the physiotherapist on the first attendance for gait re-education and subsequently at regular intervals.

The patient's skin must be checked before and after each session; this is particularly important if the patient is having chemotherapy or radio-therapy. There may be a variance of body weight which for such a large amputation will have a direct bearing on the fit of the socket.

The component parts of the prosthesis are then examined so that their method of operation is understood by the physiotherapist; the shoe is also checked to ensure it is the one for which the prosthesis was made.

Socket

With the patient standing and suitably undressed, the physiotherapist should check the socket for the following:

— The iliac crests are accommodated within the socket
— The ischial weightbearing area is correctly positioned: i.e. for the hemipelvectomy, on the ischium and buttock of the sound side; for the hip disarticulation, on the ischium of the amputated side
— The socket contains the pelvis with no excess flesh over the brim of the socket and no obvious gaps between the socket walls and the patient
— The patient is wearing suitable underclothes (see p.109) and a pair of shoes.

Once the check of the fit of the socket is complete with the patient standing, it should be checked with the patient sitting:

— The upper brim of the socket should not bite into the flesh of an obese patient
— The upper brim of the socket should not make contact with the lower ribs

— The gluteal and perineal areas should be comfortable
— The foam cosmetic covering of the prosthesis should not restrict flexion of the knee joint:

Problems that may be encountered with the socket

Socket too large

There may be excessive movement between the socket and the patient's tissues. This may be tested by asking the patient to take weight through the remaining leg and lift the prosthesis. If the prosthesis drops excessively then the socket is too large. (This is important because the socket provides suspension for the prosthesis in addition to containing the tissues.) Gaps between the socket and the patient's tissues, and excessively rubbed areas on the patient's skin, are also indications that the socket is too large.

The physiotherapist should check:

— That the prosthesis has been correctly applied
— That the fastenings are as tight as necessary for a snug fit
— Whether the patient has lost weight
— What underwear is worn.

If the socket is too large the physiotherapist must telephone the prosthetist for an urgent appointment and must not add pads or sponges to alter the socket.

Socket too small

There will be rolls of flesh over the brim of the socket, which will be excessively uncomfortable, especially when the patient sits. In addition, the patient's pelvis may not be contained within the socket; this will be particularly noticeable on the lateral aspect of the amputated side. The fastenings will be at their full length.

If the socket appears too small, the physiotherapist should check:

— That the prosthesis has been correctly applied
— That the fastenings cannot be released further
— Whether the patient has put on weight
— What underwear is worn.

If the socket is too small the physiotherapist must telephone the prosthetist for an urgent appointment.

Suspension

As the suspension is maintained by the socket, correct fit of the socket is essential. Auxiliary suspension in the form of a shoulder strap is required by some patients. This is placed over the opposite shoulder to the amputated side and should be adjusted to a firm suspension when the patient is standing.

Length

The prosthesis is made to the natural leg length. Adjustment can be made at the fitting stage to ensure a safe and smooth swing through, depending on the ability of the patient.

Prosthesis too long

The physiotherapist should check:

— The fit of the socket
— That the shoes are a pair
— The posture of the patient (some patients acquire a postural abnormality and pelvic drop with these high level amputations)
— That suspension of the prosthesis is maintained.

As a temporary measure a raise can be added to the shoe of the remaining foot. The length should be checked by the prosthetist as soon as possible.

Prosthesis too short

The physiotherapist should check:

— The fit of the socket
— That the shoes are a pair
— The posture of the patient.

As a temporary measure a raise can be added to the shoe on the prosthetic foot. The prosthesis must be checked by the prosthetist as soon as possible.

Alignment

The prosthesis will have been aligned by the prosthetist to give stability during the stance phase so that the amputee can control the hip, knee and foot mechanisms. When viewed from the lateral side the knee of the prosthesis appears hyperextended (Fig. 10.4).

If the alignment of the prosthesis appears incorrect, i.e. the patient feels unstable during the stance phase or there is an uneven swing phase of the prosthesis, the physiotherapist should check:

— The fit of the socket
— That firm suspension is maintained
— That the patient has not changed the shoes (i.e. altered the height of the heel)
— That the length of the prosthesis is correct.

The physiotherapist should contact the prosthetist if it is felt that the alignment is incorrect.

FUNCTIONAL RE-EDUCATION WITH THE PROSTHESIS

Patients with hemipelvectomy or hip disarticulation amputation regain their balance easily. Much of their rehabilitation depends on the confidence and experience of the physiotherapist, as psychological adjustment and acceptance of the large cumbersome prosthesis, slow gait and certain lack of speed of function, (e.g. turning round, sitting, climbing stairs or inclines) forms the larger part of their prosthetic rehabilitation.

Patients with these levels of amputation do not wear stump socks. The sockets of their prostheses give a large amount of tissue support and the patient's skin often becomes hot and sweaty. Therefore during treatment the prosthesis should be removed several times to check the skin condition. It is important that smooth cotton underwear with no seams or creases is used to prevent this. A long vest, smooth cotton pants or a body stocking are all suitable. However, it is often difficult to persuade a child or teenager not to wear nylon briefs and to wear long cotton vests.

The patient should be given short, clear instructions at all stages of functional re-education. Competence in the use of the prosthesis is more quickly achieved if each stage is taken in turn.

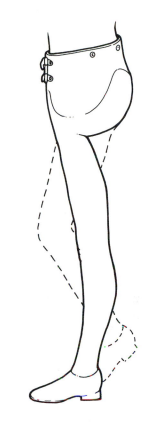

Fig. 10.4   Correct alignment of the hip disarticulation prosthesis. This permits the groung reaction force to pass anterior to the knee causing an extension moment and thus stability during the stance phase.

Application (see Fig.10.5)

The patient must learn to put on the prosthesis independently.
1. Stand, back against a wall, with bars, frame or furniture at either side.
2. Suitable underwear must be worn.
3. Grasp the socket of the prosthesis and thrust the pelvis laterally into the socket. The prosthesis should be slightly laterally rotated at this stage.
4. The pelvis must be in total contact with all the socket.
5. Fasten the straps of the socket; this will slightly medially rotate the prosthesis.
6. The shoulder strap, if used, should be secured and adjusted whilst still standing.

Removal

1. Stand and unfasten the straps.

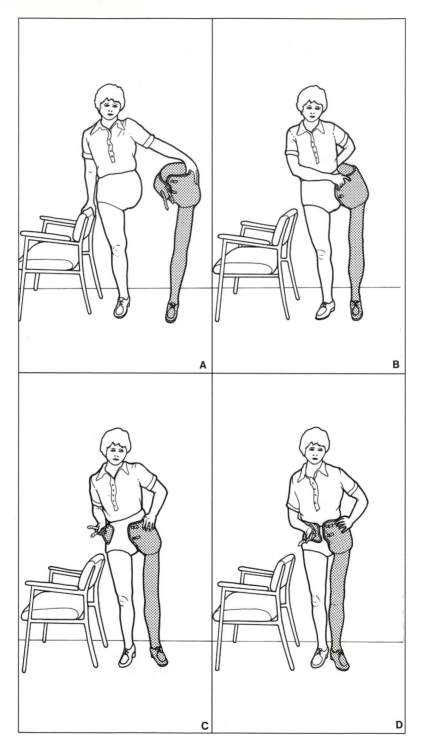

Fig. 10.5   Application of the hip disarticulation prosthesis.

2. Remove the prosthesis by grasping the socket and easing the pelvis away from it.
3. Examine the skin for any redness, rubbing or spots. A mirror may be needed to view posteriorly.

Dressing

1. Dress the prosthesis first (if trousers are being worn).
2. Place remaining leg through trousers.
3. Apply prosthesis.
4. Check the shoes are a pair and are the same shoes for which the prosthetic foot was measured.
5. Dress the top half of the body.

If must be remembered that the socket will increase the size of the amputee's pelvis. This must be taken into account when buying clothes.

Toilet

Men manage to stand and urinate with few problems wearing their prosthesis.

It is often uncomfortable to sit on a lavatory seat and inconvenient to remove underwear, so most patients, particularly women, have to remove their prosthesis before using the lavatory.

Standing from a chair

1. Push up using both hands and the remaining leg.
2. Stand erect, thrusting pelvis forward.
3. Manually lock the knee mechanism (if one is present).

Sitting down

This is more difficult than standing and walking. It may be necessary at first for patients to practise without clothes on, so that they can visualise the release.

Sitting down with Canadian joint with hip limiter (Fig. 10.6)

1. The patient should stand erect with hip neutral in order to release the limiter mechanism. The button or lever must be maintained in the release position, otherwise it will latch again in extension. The buttocks should be

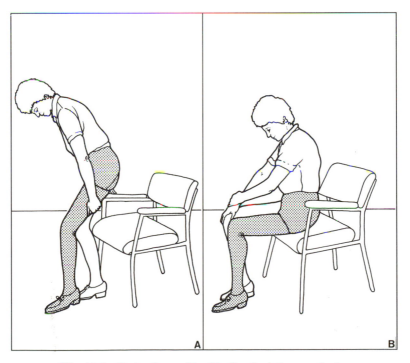

Fig. 10.6   Sitting down with a hip disarticulation prosthesis.

thrust backwards and the trunk bent forwards with both knees flexed in order to sit. The thigh section may need pushing forward with the hand (see Fig. 10.6).
2. If no lock is present the patient should lean backwards slightly to release the hip limiter, then push the thigh section forward with the hand in order to sit.

Sitting down with the four-bar linkage and joints without limiters

The patient should tilt the pelvis backwards, extend the lumbar spine, then flex the hip in order to sit. This flowing S-shaped movement takes practice and the patient needs to sit with a purposeful action.

Standing exercise

For this exercise the patient stands with feet approximately 15 cm apart. The physiotherapist should teach the following:

1. Hip hitching (this may not be possible with the hemipelvectomy level).
2. Pelvic tilt, or flick.
3. A combination of hip hitching and pelvic tilt.
4. Stepping forwards with remaining leg.
5. Hitching, pelvic tilt and initiation of the swing of prosthesis from toe off to heel strike.

The patient should not have too long a step initially in order to achieve stability when first learning to use the prosthesis. The length of the stride in the moving hip mechanisms can be altered by the prosthetist if required. Some experienced limb wearers may be taught by their prosthetists how to lengthen their stride by altering the hip limiter adjustment.

Walking

The physiotherapist should:
1. Encourage small and equal steps and emphasise weightbearing through the prosthesis by encouraging the patient to step forwards with the remaining leg first. It is sometimes difficult to transfer weight through the prosthesis at first as the patient is so used to hopping on the remaining leg.

2. During the stance phase, encourage the patient to use the back extensor muscles and the hip extensors of the remaining leg in order to maintain an erect trunk posture. This is to prevent excessive movement of the upper trunk and shoulders during the gait cycle.

3. Discourage vaulting on the remaining leg. However, some hemipelvectomy patients are unable to prevent this, and all amputees of these levels will vault to some extent in order to gain momentum and for ground clearance.

Walking aids

Once the amputee has mastered a three- or two-point gait pattern in the parallel bars and can sit down and stand up, progression to walking aids is made.

In spite of the large prosthesis, the amputee learns to control the joint components easily, usually progressing to walking sticks. This can be commenced using one stick and one bar and then progressing to two sticks within the bars. Patients usually use one stick within approximately 1 week, if attending daily for treatment.

One of the problems patients discover using their prosthesis is that their walking speed is slow. This is especially true of the young amputee who is speedy and mobile when hopping using elbow crutches. This has to be recognised by the physiotherapist and discussed. It is important that patients realise that although they are faster on crutches, there is less independence using two hands for propulsion, and standing on one leg for a length of time is tiring. It may be more desirable for the amputee's comfort and posture to stand on two legs.

Activities of daily living

Functional activity is the most relevant form of gait re-education for high level amputees, both within the home and outside in the local environment.

Walking on different surfaces

This must be practised both inside and outside the hospital under the supervision of a therapist, linoleum, different thicknesses of carpet, pavement, grass, gravel and rough ground must all be attempted. The amputee must be confident on these surfaces both alone and when outside in crowded situations, e.g. busy streets, shops, etc.

Different surfaces will transmit different sensations up through the socket. The patient must learn to recognise these new feelings and adapt accordingly. The amount of hitching and pelvic tilt required during the swing phase of the prosthesis will be different for each surface, and balance reactions will be varied.

Stairs

The same method for climbing stairs is used here as for the above-knee amputees (Ch. 11, p.128). The remaining leg goes up first and the prosthesis down first.

Step/kerb

Again, when the amputee is negotiating steps the remaining leg goes up first and the prosthesis down first (Ch. 11, p. 129).

Ramps/hills

It is advisable that if a knee-locking mechanism is present, it is locked when descending a gradient. When the patient becomes a more experienced limb user, the knee may be released.

The remaining leg leads when going uphill and the prosthesis is hitched up level with the remaining foot. When descending, the sticks are placed forwards first, followed by the prosthesis, and then the remaining foot is brought level with the prosthetic foot (see Ch. 11, p. 129).

When the gradient is steep, patients using the Canadian tilting table prosthesis must learn to control the movement of the hip and maintain it in extension during the stance phase on descending. If there are problems with descending ramps it may be that the prosthetic foot does not have a soft enough action. Flat shoes are a distinct advantage.

Whilst the amputee should obviously be taught the skills to cope with gradients, ramps are not necessarily helpful for them. Stair climbing with an adjacent handrail is often much easier.

Getting up from the floor

It is rare that patients with these levels of amputation fall, as their cadence is slow and they are careful and controlled when walking. However, they may choose to sit on the floor and should therefore practise getting up.

Method 1 (see Fig. 10.7)

1. Lie supine and gather the walking sticks (if used).
2. Release hip lock if present and sit up.
3. Lock knee mechanism if present.
4. Roll over, leading with prosthesis, onto natural knee.
5. Unlock knee mechanism so that you are kneeling on both knees.
6. Push up on both hands, or use sticks and remaining leg to steady.
7. Stand upright.

Method 2 (see Fig. 10.8)

This is the same as Method 1 except a chair can be used to push up from.

PROSTHESES INFORMATION

Detailed information regarding prostheses available in the UK can be obtained from the manufacturers. The addresses are listed in the Appendix.

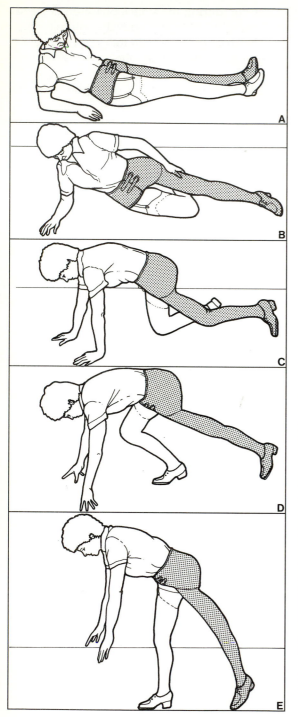

Fig. 10.7   The hip disarticulation amputee getting up from the floor. Method 1.

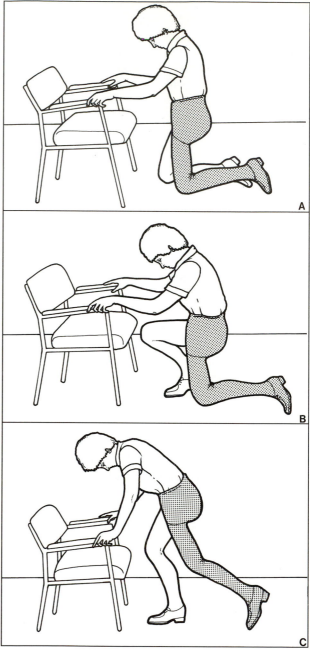

Fig. 10.8   The hip disarticulation amputee getting up from the floor using a chair. Method 2.

REFERENCES

Shurr D G, Cok T M, Buckwalter J A, Cooper R R 1983 Hip disarticulation: A prosthetic follow-up. Orthotics and Prosthetics 37(3): 50–57

van der Waarde T 1984 Ottawa experience with hip disarticulation prostheses. Orthotics and Prosthetics 38(1): 29–35

Walders J D, Davis B C 1979 Prosthetic fitting and points of rehabilitation for hindquarter and hip disarticulation patients. Physiotherapy 65(1): 4–6

11. The above-knee level of amputation

The above-knee level is a common level of amputation; its great advantage is that for the vascular patient complete healing occurs in a short space of time. This means that the patient can be discharged home quickly with few surgical complications. There is a higher mortality rate at this level than for more distal levels and the patient will have to cope with an artificial knee joint, which is energetic work: on average 49% more mean oxygen consumption than normal. It is not a suitable level of amputation for children, as the lower epiphyseal plate is removed and the stump does not grow with the child.

It is possible to fit a prosthesis to a very short stump, but the muscle control and leverage is greater with a longer stump and the prosthetist will find it easier to give the patient a more functional prosthesis. There must, however, be a gap of at least 13 cm between the distal end of the stump and the natural knee joint line. This allows enough space for an artificial knee component and permits excellent cosmesis.

It is also possible to accommodate a moderate amount of fixed flexion at the hip, but this will not permit a natural gait pattern; the cosmesis tends to be poor and at times unacceptable.

For each patient there will be an individual acceptable degree of fixed hip flexion, dependent upon body proportions, flexibility of the lumbar spine and importance of function and cosmesis. For these reasons it is difficult to state specific angles; however, approximately 25° hip flexion can be accommodated within the prosthesis. It is still possible to make a prosthesis with between 25° and 50° hip flexion, but the thigh section will obviously protrude making dressing difficult.

SOCKETS

Conventional socket

This socket has an ill-defined shape but allows weightbearing both through an ischial seating area and through the brim and walls of the socket. This is often termed the 'plug fit'. This variety of socket suits both the obese patient who has a shapeless stump and the patient with a short flexed stump. It is generally supplied only as a replacement socket for an established limb wearer.

Quadrilateral and Health (H-type) sockets

Although these sockets vary slightly, they have a similar design which allows transmission of most of the body weight through the ischial seating. Their shape prevents the stump slipping downwards giving the 'plug-fit'. In both sockets the anterior and lateral walls are sufficiently high to maintain the tissues over the posterior weightbearing area. However, during stance phase the hip abductors pull the distal femur against the lateral wall of the socket, causing the ischial tuberosity to move medially along the socket seat.

In the quadrilateral socket (see Fig. 11.1), weight is taken on the posterior brim of the socket. In the H-type socket, weight is taken on the posteromedial brim of the socket.

Ischial ramus containment (IRC) socket

This is an intimately fitting socket containing the ischial ramus and fitting to within $\frac{1}{2}$ in of the anus. It has been evolving since the late 1970s after its invention by John Sabolich in Oklahoma.

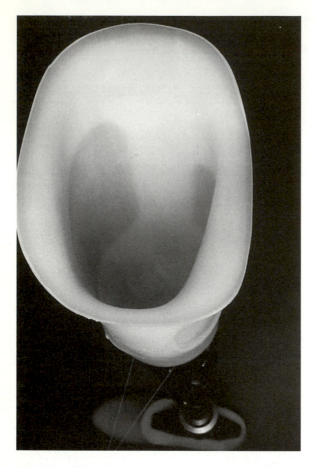

Fig. 11.1   The quadrilateral socket shape. (Reproduced from Redhead et al 1991.)

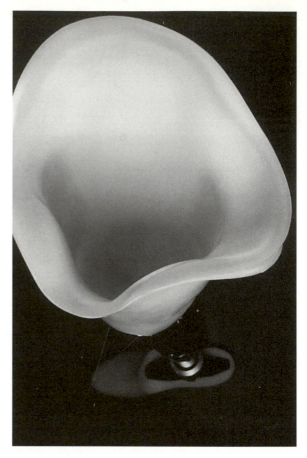

Fig. 11.2   The ischeal ramus containment socket shape. (Reproduced from Redhead et al 1991.)

It has also been known as the CAT–CAM socket (contour adducted trochanteric/controlled alignment method). The casting procedure requires specific skills of the prosthetist and may take longer than that for other sockets.

The socket itself is contoured around the skeleton and muscle groups, relying on a total contact fit for its weightbearing (see Fig. 11.2). There is a high lateral wall extending above the greater trochanter of the femur. Because of the high medial wall the ischial tuberosity is locked in the socket. The femur is held in marked adduction preventing lateral femoral shift. Weight is taken on the shaped subtrochanteric area as well as throughout the socket.

The suction socket

The patient's weight is taken mainly through the ischial seating area and tissue support is given by the walls of the socket. There is no distal support and there is a small gap between the distal end of the stump and the valve causing a negative pressure; thus there is a likelihood of congestion forming in the distal tissues. The valve permits a two-way air flow, and the method of application of this socket creates sufficient vacuum to maintain suspension with the aid of active muscle contraction in the stump. The valve is either a screw-in or push fit design. Occasionally, auxiliary suspension is required.

Total surface bearing (TSB) sockets

These sockets are made of various plastic materials with recently developed new flexible properties.

The patient's weight is taken through the whole socket as well as the ischial weightbearing area. The stump tissues are in contact with all aspects of the socket; the fit is extremely accurate and a stump sock is not worn. The valve permits only a one-way flow of air outwards from the socket. This exclusion of air, as well as the active contraction of the stump muscles, maintains the suspension of the prosthesis. There is no negative pressure; therefore the distal tissues are supported. Occasionally, auxiliary suspension, such as a Silesian belt, may be required.

These last three sockets are given to patients with stable mature stumps, good muscle control, full hip joint mobility, no oedema and no gross scarring.

The advantages of these sockets are that:

a. through the intimate contact with the patient's skin, sensory feedback is enhanced
b. muscle contraction provides an instant prosthetic movement, with no time lapse or pistoning.

Materials used in above-knee socket fabrication

Plastics. The vast majority of sockets for this level are made of plastic. They can be manufactured rapidly, are simple to replace and are easy to clean. The disadvantage is that they are rather hot to wear. Some plastics are both flexible and soft (e.g. Surlyn) and can provide a socket within a rigid support frame (e.g. the ISNY socket, see Fig. 7.3).

Metal. This material is still used for sockets as it has the advantages of being easily adjustable and cool to wear, and the socket may have ventilation holes cut.

Wood. This material is used for hot climates as it is comfortable to wear and easy for a carpenter to learn to fashion, particularly in less developed countries where technology and industry are not as sophisticated as in the industrial market economies of the West.

SUSPENSION

Rigid pelvic band (RPB) (see Fig. 11.7)

This fits snugly around the contours of the pelvis. There is a uniaxial joint between the RPB and its attachment to the lateral brim of the socket which allows for only flexion and extension of the hip joint. In the majority of cases a shoulder strap over the contralateral shoulder gives additional support.

Soft suspension

This needs to be adjusted when standing. Therefore good balance, hand grip and hand–eye coordination are necessary.

Roehampton soft suspension (RSS) (see Fig. 11.3)

This is a leather waist belt with two diagonal down straps to the anterior and lateral sides of the socket. A well-defined waist is needed.

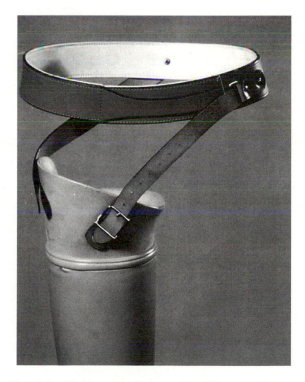

Fig. 11.3 Roehampton soft suspension. (Photograph by kind permission of C. A. Blatchford & Sons Ltd.)

Silesian belt

This is a simple wrap-around strap connected to the anterior and lateral sides of the socket. It is usually used as an auxiliary suspension for a suction or self-suspending socket.

Total elastic suspension (TES) (see Fig. 11.4)

This is made of Neoprene and can be hot to wear. It does not control rotation of the prosthesis or lateral drift of the socket.

Fashioned belts

There are other designs individually fashioned for women or the elderly, which employ shaped waist belts and vertical elastic downstraps.

KNEE COMPONENTS

Stance phase controls

Semi-automatic knee lock (SAKL)

This is a spring-loaded mechanism which automatically locks in extension. There is a manual control to release it so that the knee is flexed when sitting. This is the simplest knee mechanism available. It is also the safest knee mechanism and therefore most suitable for the unsteady or geriatric patient.

Stabilised knee

This design is advantageous to all patients capable of using a moving knee, as it gives total stability for up to 22° flexion at the knee joint during stance phase, and is a free swinging knee in swing

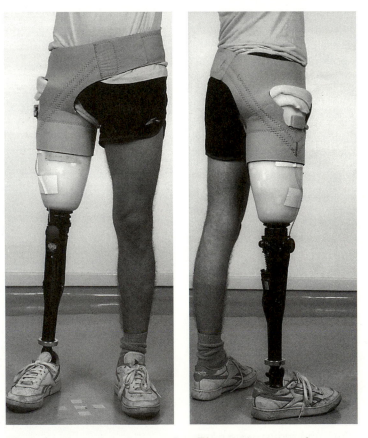

Fig. 11.4   The total elastic suspension. (Photograph courtesy of Richmond, Twickenham & Roehampton Health Authority Medical Photography Department.)

phase. Its design is particularly useful for patients walking on rough ground or descending hills, ramps, etc. The range of stability allowed can be altered only by the prosthetist. To test this stabilising mechanism, the physiotherapist should remove the prosthesis from the patient, hold the socket and push manually and vertically downwards to the forefoot, with the knee slightly flexed. If the knee remains fixed in this position while weight is being applied the stabilising mechanism is present. This design can be supplied with a hand-operated knee lock (HOKL) if required.

There is also a stance-flex component which

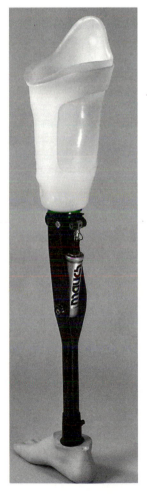

Fig. 11.5   The Mauch Swing 'n Stance Knee unit on an above-knee prosthesis with an ischeal ramus containment socket. (Photograph by kind permission of C. A. Blatchford & Sons Ltd.)

permits some controlled flexion at heel contact. It gives additional shock absorption and enhanced performance and is particularly useful for the active patient.

Four-bar linkage

This joint is inherently stable for up to about 12° of knee flexion during the stance phase and is a free swinging knee during swing phase. This mechanism is illustrated in Figures 10.1 and 10.3. The design is especially suitable for the very long above-knee stump.

Swing phase controls

These components will control the rate of swing of the lower leg during swing phase, depending on the muscle action of the stump and the forward momentum of the amputee.

Pneumatic control (i.e. air control) will adjust to variations of gait cadence in a limited range.

Hydraulic control (i.e. fluid control) has a broad range of variation to gait cadence. Examples are the Mauch and Otto Bock units. There are separate adjustment valves for flexion control and extension control (see Fig. 11.5).

Wheel-type knee control and extension bias aids are simple swing phase controls found on older style prostheses.

FOOT COMPONENTS

For details of these, see Chapter 7 (p. 76).

CHECK OF THE ABOVE-KNEE PROSTHESIS

The fit of the prosthesis should be checked by the physiotherapist on the first attendance for gait re-education, and subsequently at regular intervals. The patient's ability to function with the prosthesis will depend upon a correct fit.

There may have been an interval of time between the delivery of the prosthesis and this first attendance, and the patient's body and stump may have changed in shape and size. The patient should always be suitably undressed for this procedure.

Socket

Quadrilateral and H-type sockets

1. Ischial seating

To check that the ischial tuberosity is correctly placed on the socket, the patient should stand with all the weight on the remaining leg. The physiotherapist locates the ischial tuberosity of the affected side with the palmar aspect of two fingers and then asks the patient to transfer weight on to the prosthesis. Full contact should be felt with the fingers between the patient's ischial tuberosity and the seating area of the socket. If the ischial tuberosity slides down inside, the socket is too large. If the tuberosity is above the seating area, the socket is too small.

Socket too large: the physiotherapist can add more stump socks of a variety of thicknesses.

Socket too small: the physiotherapist can decrease the number and thickness of the socks.

If the above measures do not correct the fit of the socket, the physiotherapist should telephone the prosthetist and request an appointment for adjustments to be made.

2. The adductor region

There should be no discomfort in this sensitive area. If the patient reports discomfort:

— Check that the patient is not 'sinking' into the socket and that there is correct weightbearing through the ischial tuberosity.
— Check that the stump socks are well pulled up over the rim of the socket.
— Check for fixed flexion contracture in the affected hip and compare this with the set of the socket.
— Check the strength and function of the hip extensor muscles on the affected side.
— With the patient standing correctly observe the adductor flare of the socket. This may need adjustment by the prosthetist.

3. The distal end of the stump

No discomfort should be experienced in this area. If an area of redness appears on the anterior aspect of the distal end of the stump, the patient may have a fixed flexion contracture of the hip which is not adequately accommodated in the socket.

If oedema occurs in the distal end of the stump, the patient may need soft tissue support by means of a soft pad, or the socket may be too narrow causing interruption of lymphatic and venous return. For either of these problems, the physiotherapist should telephone the prosthetist.

IRC and self-suspending sockets

These sockets can feel very hard to the patient initially and the tissues of the stump have to become accustomed to them.

The problems that can occur are discomfort and a feeling of lack of suspension. This is because the interface between the stump and the socket is incorrect: the socket is too tight, too loose, or the method of application is incorrect.

The physiotherapist can check the patient's weight, general health and ability to don the prosthesis; the prosthetist then needs to be contacted if none of the above are contributing factors.

Length

To check the length of the prosthesis the physiotherapist stands behind the patient, hands resting on the patient's iliac crests. The patient should be suitably undressed so that the whole spine can be observed for rotation and scoliosis. The iliac crests should be approximately level when the patient is standing with equal weight on both legs.

The more important check of the length of the prosthesis is in the dynamic situation when walking. The patient must have safe clearance of the foot from the floor without producing gait abnormalities.

If the prosthesis is too long the physiotherapist should check that:

— The patient is wearing two shoes which are a pair
— The remaining knee is not held in flexion
— The socket is not too small so that the stump is being pushed up out of the socket.

If the prosthesis still appears to be too long, an adjustable sandal shoe raise (Fig. 11.6) can be

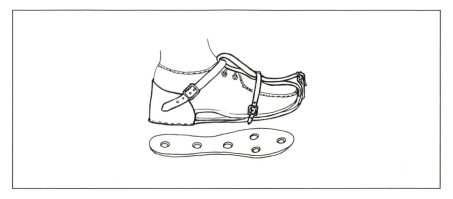

Fig. 11.6 An adjustable sandal shoe raise. Extra insoles, like the one shown, may be added between the patient's shoe and the sandal until the correct leg length is obtained.

used to accurately assess the length discrepancy. A temporary cork shoe raise can then be stuck on the shoe of the remaining leg.

If the prosthesis is too short, the physiotherapist should check that:

— The shoes are a pair
— The socket is not too large.

Again it is possible to use the adjustable sandal on the shoe of the prosthesis to assess any necessary cork raise required. In either case it is advisable to telephone the prosthetist for length adjustment.

Suspension

Rigid pelvic band (RPB) suspension

This should fit snugly around the contours of the pelvis. If there is discomfort here:

— Check the clothing that is worn between the RPB and the skin
— Remove and re-apply the prosthesis.

However, if the discomfort persists, the set and position of the RPB will need adjusting. An incorrectly set RPB can also cause medial or lateral rotation of the prosthesis.

Shoulder strap

The tension of the shoulder strap must be checked with the patient standing. If it is too tight it will tend to make the patient stoop forwards. If it is too loose it will not contribute adequately to the suspension.

Soft suspension

With the patient suitably undressed, the physiotherapist should check that the waist or Silesian belt is of the correct tension and the downstraps are correctly angled and also under correct tension when the patient is standing and walking.

With the TES belt, the physiotherapist should check that it has been wrapped around the pelvis correctly and that it has been fastened with the correct tension anteriorly.

Knee mechanism

The physiotherapist should check the working of the knee mechanism to ensure that it stabilises, flexes and (if a lock is present) that it locks and releases efficiently. The patient should fully understand the theory of the function of the knee components supplied.

FUNCTIONAL RE-EDUCATION WITH THE PROSTHESIS

The patient should be given short, clear instructions at all stages of functional re-education. Competence in the use of the prosthesis is more quickly achieved if each stage is taken in turn.

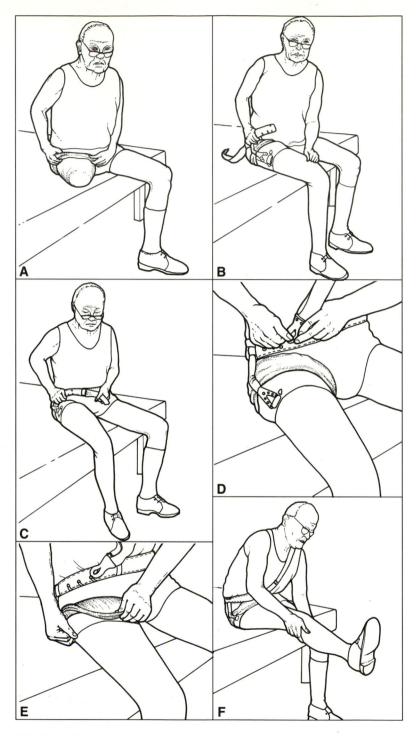

Fig. 11.7   Application of the above-knee temporary prosthesis with RPB.

Application

Rigid pelvic band (see Fig. 11.7)

This is the only prosthesis that can be applied easily while sitting down.

1. Sit on a firm bed, undressed apart from a vest.
2. Pull the stump sock smoothly up over the stump (Fig. 11.7A).
3. With the knee joint of the prosthesis flexed and the foot in lateral rotation, slide the stump into the socket (Fig. 11.7B)
4. Fasten the RPB loosely over the vest (Fig. 11.7C).
5. The shoulder strap (if used) should be fastened when sitting and adjusted for height when standing (Fig. 11.7D).
6. Pull the stump sock up and out over the rim of the socket to prevent wrinkling (Fig. 11.7E). This position can be maintained with a large safety pin securing the sock around the metal upright of the hip joint.
7. Lock the knee in extension, then stand up with the aid of rails or a frame (Fig. 11.7F).
8. Fasten the RPB securely. This will rotate the foot into the correct mid-position.

Some patients with good balance can slide the stump, with the sock on, into the socket of the prosthesis while they are standing. The knee joint should be locked and the prosthesis laterally rotated before the RPB is secured.

Soft suspension

The prosthesis may be applied to the stump with the patient sitting, but fastening of the suspension can only be done with the patient standing. Excellent standing balance is required without hand holds, but the patient may need to lean against a wall or sturdy furniture. The critical application of the angle of the straps and the correct tension of the waist/pelvic band must be understood by both physiotherapist and patient. If there are any problems the prosthetist should be contacted concerning the correct detail.

Self-suspending sockets

The patient is first taught how to apply this type of socket by the prosthetist. It is difficult for the physiotherapist to assist the patient other than by encouraging the correct coordination of this procedure and providing time to practise.

The patient must have good coordination, standing balance and great patience, particularly during the first few weeks, in order to be successful.

The basic wrap method (see Fig. 11.8)

Some patients may prefer to use a stump sock or a silk scarf instead of a bandage. The amputee is instructed to:

1. Stand up, with either a chair or the wall behind, and with the prosthesis resting close by.
2. Using a 15 cm wide Elset or crepe bandage, lightly bandage the stump with 2–3 turns (according to length of the stump) from medial to lateral, starting posteriorly and proximally (Fig. 11.8A).
3. Make a tuck with the long end of the bandage into the anterior distal twin turns, fixing the bandage to the stump and leaving a long portion free (Fig. 11.8B).
4. Feed the long end of the bandage inside the socket and pull it out through the valve hole (Fig. 11.8C).
5. Place the stump inside the socket with the prosthesis in correct alignment.
6. Gradually withdraw the bandage through the valve hole, gently drawing the stump tissue down into the socket (Fig. 11.8D). During this procedure, gently ease the stump downwards into the socket. Should the bandage become stuck at any stage, find the approximate position and stop withdrawing the bandage; this allows time for the stump tissues to move. If possible, ease the stump away from the offending area, then resume withdrawing the bandage by pulling on each edge alternately.
7. The whole bandage should be pulled out through the valve hole. The stump should be correctly positioned in the socket at this stage; there should be no space between the stump and the valve with the TSB socket, but there

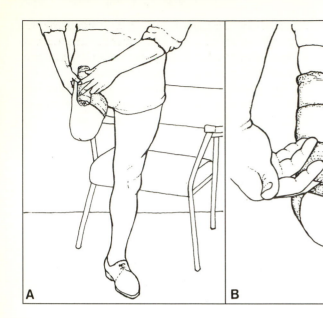

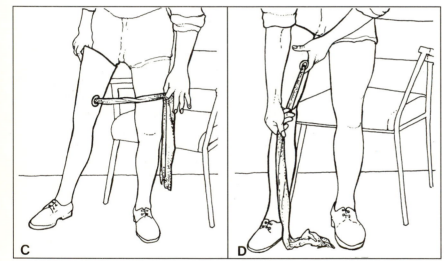

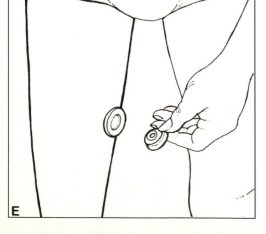

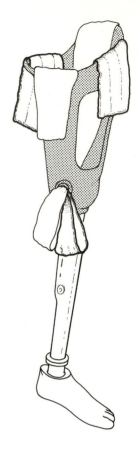

Fig. 11.9 The four-loop method showing the starting position of the two draped bandages.

Fig. 11.8 Application of the suction socket by the wrap method.

should be a small gap of approximately 2 cm with the suction socket.

8. Locate the valve in the valve hole (Fig. 11.8E).

The four-loop method

This is another method of application of the self-suspending socket (Fig. 11.9). Two 10 cm wide Elset bandages are used in the positions shown. Four lengths are draped over the anterior, posterior, medial and lateral aspects of the brim of the socket: the length draped is determined by the patient by practice, but it is at least as long as the stump. The patient stands in narrow stride standing, with the remaining leg in front. The stump is pushed into the socket as far as it will go and then the bandage is drawn out through the valve hole, a little at a time. This will ease in each section of the stump at a time.

The wrap method will only ease the tissues in from the top of the circumference of the stump, whereas this method will ease in the buttock tissues as well and is the only method for the IRC socket. This method is also useful for amputees with fluctuating stump volume as it is a more rigorous method of drawing the tissues into the socket.

Dressing

The patient should be instructed to:

1. Pull the underpants and trousers (if worn) up over the prosthesis before applying it to the stump.
2. Apply the prosthesis.
3. Slot the remaining leg into the underpants and trousers, then fasten over the suspension. If underpants or knickers are worn inside the suspension, use of the lavatory is impossible. Trouser legs may need to be widened with a triangular insert in the inside leg seam, as the socket and knee components may be broader than the natural limb.
4. Check that the same shoe (or shoe of similar heel height) is on the prosthesis. This is because the artificial foot is aligned for one height of heel. Check also that the matching shoe is on the remaining leg.

5. Dress the top half of the body in the normal way. The shoulder strap should be underneath the shirt/blouse.

Undressing

All patients can do this seated, but those with excellent standing balance may prefer to remove the prosthesis while standing.

First, the suspension should be unfastened, the socket eased off the stump and the stump sock (if worn) removed.

Second, all patients should be taught to inspect the stump routinely for any areas of redness, rubbing or spots. A mirror may be needed to view the posterior and medial aspects of the stump.

Toilet

1. For a man standing to urinate, there are no problems.
2. Good balance is necessary for the removal of clothing prior to sitting down; grab rails may be needed in the early stages of rehabilitation.
3. When sitting, patients may prefer to abduct the hips to prevent soiling of the stump sock and medial edge of the socket.
4. Some patients may prefer to remove their prosthesis before going to the toilet (particularly women).

GAIT RE-EDUCATION IN THE ABOVE-KNEE PROSTHESIS

The physiotherapist must check the fit of the prosthesis before gait re-education. The patient should always start in the parallel bars.

It is important that regular strengthening and mobility exercises are maintained during this phase of rehabilitation.

The procedures for initial gait re-education and progression to walking aids is described in detail in Chapter 9. In order for successful, smooth gait to be achieved by the above-knee amputee, both the patient and the physiotherapist must understand the properties of the knee component supplied. Individual gait training will therefore vary.

Walking on different surfaces

This must be practised both indoors and outside under the supervision of the physiotherapist. Linoleum, different thicknesses of carpet, pavement, grass, gravel and rough ground must all be attempted. The amputee must be confident on these surfaces both alone and when outside in crowded situations.

Different surfaces will transmit different sensations up through the socket to the stump. The patient must learn to recognise these new feelings and adapt the gait pattern accordingly. The younger patient can practise altering speed of reaction on a wobble board in the physiotherapy department (see Fig. 11.10).

Stairs

The patient is first taught to climb stairs with two bannisters. When ascending, the remaining leg leads; when descending, the prosthesis leads. The patient then progresses to using one stick and one bannister. It is very important that the patient, when descending, places the stick down one stair before stepping down with the prosthesis.

Stairs must always be practised with the physiotherapist, even if a frame is used or there are no stairs at the patient's home. The amputee's life must not be limited by immediate surroundings. If the patient walks with a frame, stairs can be managed with one stick and one bannister. If this is difficult or unsafe, then the patient faces the bannister, grasps it with both hands, and ascends and descends sideways. Two walking frames are then provided: one to keep upstairs and one downstairs.

Established users with a Mauch swing and stance control are able to descend stairs in a normal reciprocal pattern.

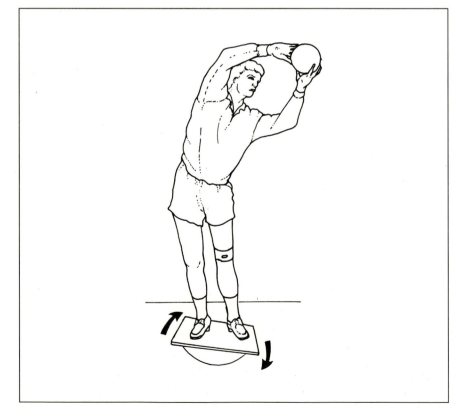

Fig. 11.10   Re-education of balance and speed of reaction using a wobble board.

Step/kerb

Unless the patient has practised negotiating steps or a kerb outside the physiotherapy department under the supervision of the physiotherapist, it is unlikely that walking outside will be achieved with confidence.

The patient should keep the feet as close to the step as possible, and step up with the remaining leg first, then step down with the prosthesis first.

Ramps and hills

These are more difficult than stairs and may be accomplished with a greater degree of safety by the patient proceeding sideways, ascending with the remaining leg first and descending with the prosthesis first.

On ascending in the forward direction, the patient must lean forwards, place the sticks well forward and lead with the remaining leg. The prosthesis should be brought level with the remaining foot.

On descending in the forward direction, the sticks are placed forwards first, then the prosthesis. The remaining foot is brought forwards parallel to the prosthetic foot.

When the gradient is steep, the hip extensor muscles of the stump must work hard to ensure balance on the prosthesis during the stance phase. The prosthetic foot is not completely in contact with the slope at this point. If the gradient is excessively steep it is always safer to ascend and descend sideways. The more able patient and those with enabling knee components may achieve equal stride lengths on slopes.

Getting up after a fall

Teaching the patient to fall down is both dangerous and unnecessary. It is the method of getting up that should be taught. The patient is always instructed to remain on the ground for a few moments after a fall to get over the shock and think out the method of recovering walking aids and getting up.

If a chair is available the patient should move across the floor either by rolling or by scooting on the buttocks, remembering to take the walking aids.

The physiotherapist should explain and demonstrate the three methods of getting up (listed below) to elderly patients. Relatives and friends are also shown these methods, and are taught correct lifting procedures if necessary. The younger fitter patients, however, practise these manoeuvres as part of their rehabilitation programme. All patients are advised on how to ask for and direct help from a member of the public who has come to their aid.

Method 1 (Fig. 11.11)

1. Turn to face the seat
2. Put both hands on the seat
3. Kneel on remaining leg with prosthesis extended behind
4. Push on hands, straighten up on remaining leg to standing
5. Release grip on chair as balance is regained and use aids.

Method 2 (Fig. 11.12)

1. Sit close to chair with back touching the seat
2. Put both hands on seat of chair
3. Flex up the knee of the remaining leg
4. Push up hard and slide both buttocks onto the seat.

Method 3 (Fig. 11.13)

This method should be used if no seat is available.

1. Gather walking aids
2. Roll prone, leading with remaining leg
3. Push up on arms and flex remaining leg
4. Start extending remaining leg, push up on one stick, regain balance, then push up on second stick.

PROSTHESES INFORMATION

Detailed information regarding prostheses available in the UK can be obtained from the manufacturers. The addresses are listed in the Appendix.

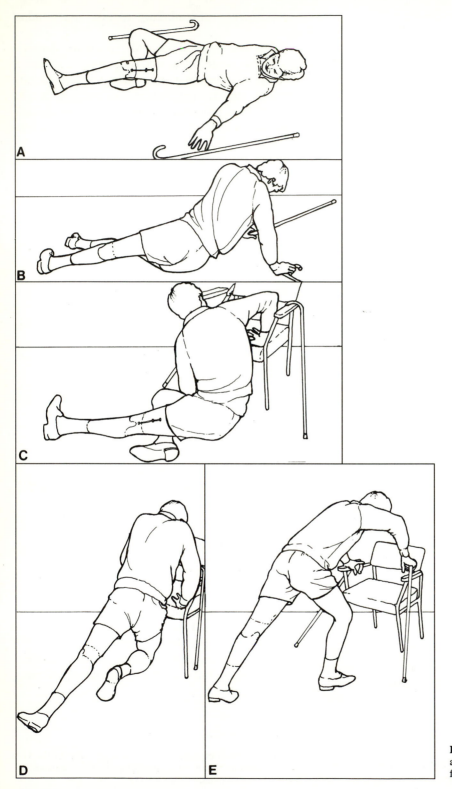

Fig. 11.11   The above-knee amputee getting up from the floor. Method 1.

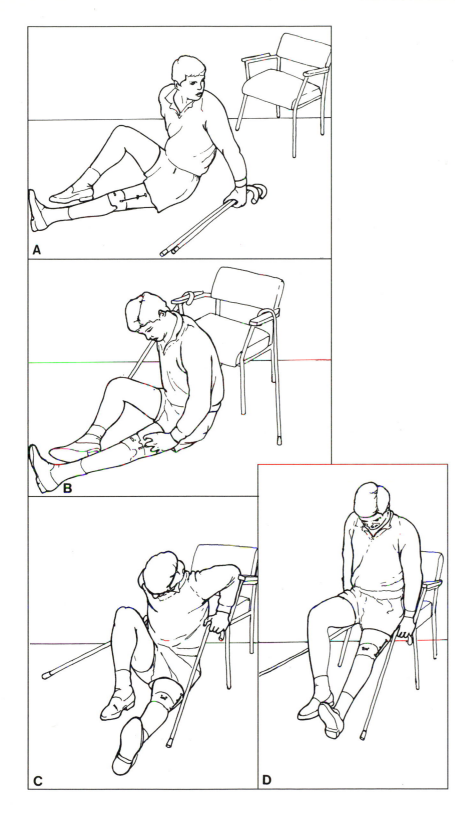

Fig. 11.12   The above-knee amputee getting up from the floor. Method 2.

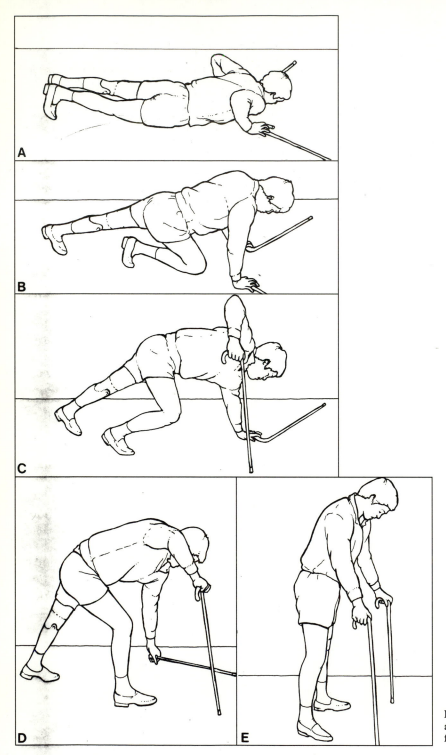

Fig. 11.13 The above-knee amputee getting up from the floor. Method 3.

REFERENCES

Gailey R, Newell C 1991 Metabolic cost of unilateral above-knee amputees walking: a comparison between the quadrilateral socket and the CAT–CAM socket. WCPT 11th International Congress Proceedings Book II: 641–643

Judge G W, Fisher L 1981 A bouncy knee for above-knee amputees. Engineering in Medicine 10 (1): 27–31

Kristinsson O 1983 Flexible above-knee socket made from low density polyethylene suspended by a weight transmitting frame. Orthotics and Prosthetics 37 (2): 25–30

Radcliffe C W 1977 The Knud Jansen Lecture. Above-knee prosthetics. Prosthetics and Orthotics International 1 (3): 146–160

Redhead R G 1979 Total surface bearing self suspending above-knee sockets. Prosthetics and Orthotics International 3 (3): 126–136

Sabolich J 1985 Contoured adducted–trochanteric controlled alignment method (CAT–CAM): introduction and principles. Clinics in Prosthetics and Orthotics 9 (4): 15–26

Schuch C M 1988 Report from: International workshop on above-knee fitting and alignment techniques. Clinical Prosthetics and Orthotics 12 (2): 81–98

Simpson D 1980 Prosthetic replacement of knee function. Physiotherapy 66 (8): 262–265

Watts H G, Carideo J F, Marich M S 1982 Variable-volume sockets for above-knee amputees. Managing children following amputation for malignancy. Inter Clinic Information Bulletin 18 (2): 11–14

12. The through-knee levels of amputation

There are four different levels of amputation about the knee joint:

1. Through-knee
2. Gritti–Stokes
3. Transcondylar
4. Supracondylar.

Through–knee

This is a disarticulation of the tibia from the femur. The patella is left in situ and the patellar tendon is sutured to the hamstring tendons and cruciate ligaments, around the end of the femur. This stump has the capability of being fully end-bearing and normal proprioception is maintained.

As all the muscles around the hip joint are intact, there is powerful control of the long lever of the stump, and its bulbous shape allows a self-suspending socket with rotational stability between socket and stump. Cosmesis has not always in the past been acceptable, particularly for women. However, lightweight endoskeletal prostheses have greatly improved the cosmesis and recent knee designs have greatly improved function.

It can be an ideal level for the elderly and also for those who may become bilateral amputees. Full weightbearing is possible both on the stumps themselves and in prostheses. Where prosthetic re-education is not possible, the long lever and endbearing properties of this level allow for good sitting balance in the wheelchair and the stump can be used as a prop when transferring.

It is also a good level for children as the distal femoral epiphysis is left intact ensuring normal growth. It can be used for the removal of a use-less congenitally deformed lower leg, e.g. phoco-melia.

This level is inadvisable if hip flexion contracture is present. In this situation the prosthesis appears bulky and is cosmetically unacceptable. Furthermore the weightbearing area may have to be transferred proximally to the ischium. This level thus becomes biomechanically the same as the above knee level, negating the endbearing properties of the stump.

Gritti–Stokes

The distal end of the femur is divided at the level of the adductor tubercle. The patella is retained, its articular surface is removed and it is sutured over the cut end of the femur. This is the classical Gritti–Stokes; however, it is rarely done.

Modified Gritti–Stokes/transcondylar

The distal end of the femur is divided at the level of the epicondyles. This is more commonly done than the classical Gritti–Stokes.

Supracondylar

The distal end of the femur is divided at about the level of the adductor tubercle. The medullary cavity is left open. This is treated as a very long above-knee amputation (see Ch. 11).

For positive confirmation of the Gritti–Stokes, transcondylar and supracondylar levels, X-rays may be required. These three levels give a stump which is a long lever with powerful hip muscle control. The bulbous end of the stump is reduced so self-suspension of the socket is not always possible and some auxiliary suspension may be required. Proprioception is lost at these levels along with some of the endbearing property of the stump, necessitating proximal weightbearing areas on the prosthesis. If the patella is retained, it frequently loosens and gives rise to pain when the patient is walking.

CONSTRUCTION OF THE THROUGH-KNEE PROSTHESIS

Sockets

Plastic socket

This is a total contact socket with a soft liner and an outer plastic hard shell. The PE Lite liner (high-density foam material) is made on a cast taken of the stump, so that the fit is intimate. The liner has a small split made in it, so that on application it will open to allow the bulbous femoral condoyles to slide through the length of the liner. When the stump touches the distal end pad, the slit closes completely.

This type of socket is usually self-suspending with the patient's weight taken totally on the distal end of the stump. If it is necessary to reduce endbearing, a proximal-bearing brim shape (e.g. quadrilateral or H-type) will need to be incorporated.

Blocked leather and metal socket

These materials are sometimes used with established limb wearers. Auxiliary suspension may also be required.

Auxiliary suspension

The three types of auxiliary suspension, namely rigid pelvic band, shoulder suspension and Silesian belt, are described in Chapter 11 and are occasionally used.

Knee mechanism

The most usual knee mechanism supplied is the four-bar linkage. Other knee mechanisms as described in Chapter 11 may also be supplied.

CHECK OF THE THROUGH-KNEE PROSTHESIS

The fit of the prosthesis should be checked by the physiotherapist on the first attendance for gait re-education and subsequently at regular intervals. The patient's function will depend on the correct fit. The patient should always be suitably undressed for this procedure.

Socket

The endbearing pad

The distal end of the stump must be supported by this pad, but the degree of weightbearing achieved will depend on the type of amputation and the stage of healing reached.

With plastic sockets it is important to check the fit of the liner on the stump, by palpating the stump through the liner; it should be a snug fit with no gaps.

If the patient reports discomfort, too much weight may be taken distally. The reasons for this may be that:

— The socket is too large
— The stump stock has formed a wrinkle between the stump and end pad
— Too much activity.

The physiotherapist may remove the end pad and insert several layers of soft foam instead, thus reducing some of the distal pressure as a temporary measure.

Another reason for discomfort may be that too little weight is taken distally and there is proximal constriction. The physiotherapist must teach the patient to watch for a cold, blue and mottled stump end, particularly on the through-knee stump.

Socket too large

If the socket is too large, pistoning and rotation will occur and suspension and alignment will be lost. This commonly happens in the early stages of prosthetic re-education as the distal stump oedema subsides and the thigh muscles atrophy. It may also happen if the patient's total weight drops by 4 kg or more.

Great care must be taken if adding more stump socks as too much pressure may be exerted over the distal condyles. The sock may be cut as a temporary measure to pad out the mid-thigh area only. Sometimes a sock added between the PE Lite liner and the hard plastic shell may create sufficient suspension as a temporary measure.

The prosthetist must be contacted for an assessment for a new liner, socket or both.

Socket too small

If the socket is too small, the stump will not slide down sufficiently to contact the endbearing pad. Constriction of the distal stump occurs and it is unlikely that the patient may function in this circumstance; 'ischaemic' stump pain may be reported.

The prosthetist must be contacted for a new liner, socket or both.

Length

Standing

A routine check of the length is made statically and dynamically (see Ch. 11).

Sitting

When the patient sits down, with with both knees flexed, the socket extends further than the natural knee. This is inevitable as the end pad and socket have to be distal to the natural knee joint line.

Auxiliary suspension

The suspension must be comfortable and secure if used (see Ch. 11).

Knee mechanism

The physiotherapist should check the working and function of the knee mechanism supplied before the patient uses the prosthesis for the first time. This will ensure that the correct method of use is taught to the patient. If there is any doubt, the physiotherapist should contact the prosthetist to check the function of the mechanism supplied.

FUNCTIONAL RE-EDUCATION WITH THE THROUGH-KNEE PROSTHESIS

The patient should be given short, clear instructions at all stages of functional re-education.

Application

The patient should be instructed as follows:

1. Sit on a firm bed and undress apart from a vest.
2. Pull the stump sock smoothly up over the stump.
3. With knee joint of the prosthesis flexed, apply the socket to the stump. The method varies according to the material of the socket.
4. After having pulled the stump sock over the stump (Fig. 12.1A), remove the PE Lite liner from the plastic shell and pull it onto the stump (Fig. 12.1B). Sometimes this procedure is difficult because the liner is such a firm fit, but the distal end of the stump must be in close contact with the foam end pad. It may be necessary to pull a nylon sock over the PE Lite liner (Fig. 12.1C) before applying the plastic socket (see Fig. 12.1D) in order to reduce friction between the two surfaces.
5. Fasten the auxiliary suspension (if present) over the vest.
6. Pull the stump sock up and out over the rim of the socket to prevent wrinkling.
7. Stand up with support, and re-adjust the suspension if necessary.

Some patients with good balance can apply the prosthesis while standing, but the knee joint of the prosthesis must be in extension.

Removal

It is simpler to remove a prosthesis than to apply it and the less able patient should attempt this first. The following instructions should be given:

1. Sit down on a firm bed or chair.
2. Undo the auxiliary suspension if present.
3. Ease the socket off the stump; the outer shell is removed first and then the PE Lite liner.
4. Remove the stump sock.

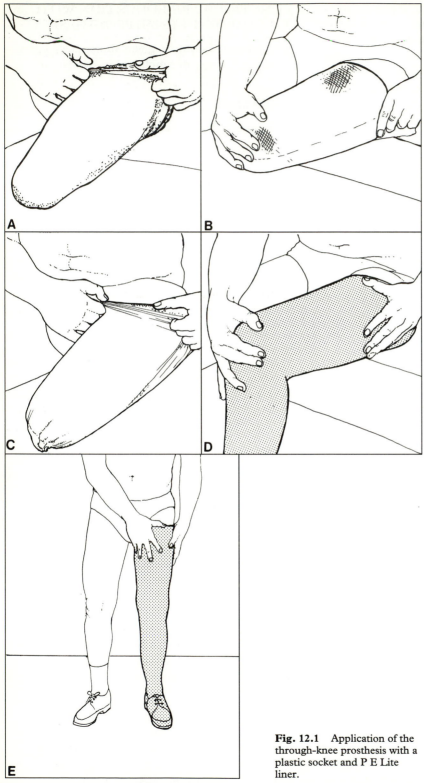

Fig. 12.1 Application of the
through-knee prosthesis with a
plastic socket and P E Lite
liner.

5. Inspect the stump thoroughly, especially the femoral condyles, for any redness, rubbing or spots. A mirror should be used to check the distal and posterior aspects.

Dressing

The same procedure is employed for patients with the through-knee level of amputation as for those with the above-knee level (see Ch. 11). However, the width of the knee of the prosthesis is maybe greater than the natural knee, so alterations to trouser leg width may be required.

Toilet

Some patients prefer not to wear the prosthesis when sitting on the toilet seat in order to have their bowels open.

GAIT RE-EDUCATION

Gait re-education is similar to that for the above-knee amputee. However, the main difference is that there is a long, powerful lever controlling the prosthesis. Smooth control of the knee mechanism and stride length using proprioception and cutaneous sensation is essential to avoid a long prosthetic stride and uneven gait pattern. Hip extensor exercises should be continued to control overactive hip flexion and resisted walking is a useful method of training.

The true through-knee amputee is able to fully weightbear through the distal end of the stump. In the prosthesis the patient with the Gritti–Stokes level of amputation may also be able to fully weightbear distally at this stage. However, if the patient complains of discomfort in the distal end of the stump, it may be that the patella has become detached from the femur and is moving as the patient walks. In this instance the physiotherapist should contact the prosthetist or the surgeon.

Patients with the modified Gritti–Stokes and supracondylar levels of amputation are never able to fully weightbear through the distal area of the stump and may have ischial weightbearing sockets. Therefore, the function is similar to the above-knee amputee.

PROSTHESES INFORMATION

Detailed information regarding prostheses available in the UK can be obtained from the manufacturers. The addresses are listed in the Appendix.

REFERENCES

Baumgartner R F 1979 Knee disarticulation versus above-knee amputation. Prosthetics and Orthotics International 3(1): 15–19

Baumgartner R F 1983 Failures in through-knee amputation. Prosthetics and Orthotics International 7:116–118

Houghton A, Allen A, Luff R, McColl I 1989 Rehabilitation after lower limb amputation: a comparative study of above-knee, through-knee and Gritti–Stokes amputations. British Journal of Surgery 76: 622–624

Jendrzejczyk D J 1980 Prosthetic management for children with knee disarticulations. Inter Clinic Information Bulletin 17(7): 9–16

Jensen J S 1983 Life expectancy and social consequences of through-knee amputations. Prosthetics and Orthotics International 7: 113–115

Jensen J S, Poulsen T M, Krasnik M 1982 Through-knee amputation. Acta Orthopaedica Scandinavica 53: 463–466

Martin P, Wickham J E A 1962 Gritti–Stokes amputation for atherosclerotic gangrene. Lancet ii: 16–17

Mensch G 1983 Physiotherapy following through-knee amputation. Prosthetics and Orthotics International 7: 79–87

Moran B J, Buttenshaw P, Mulcahy M, Robinson K P 1990 Through-knee amputation in high-risk patients with vascular disease: indications, complications and rehabilitation. British Journal of Surgery 77: 1118–1120

Thyregod H C, Holstein P, Jensen J S 1983 The healing of through-knee amputations in relation to skin perfusion pressure. Prosthetics and Orthotics International 7: 61–62

13. The below-knee level of amputation

Almost all patients will be successful prosthetic users at the below-knee level of amputation, irrespective of their physical condition or age. The knee joint is preserved, enabling the patient to gain as near normal a gait and function as is possible.

Amputees with this level consume less energy than those with higher levels, as there is a long lever controlling the prosthetic foot and ankle. It is possible to re-educate all patients with this level, provided that the correct surgical technique preserves muscle bulk and creates a good shape and scar position and that the prosthesis fits correctly and is comfortable. The patellar tendon bearing prosthesis (PTB) supplied for this level is cosmetically very acceptable and deviations from the normal gait pattern are usually undetectable. The suitable length for a below-knee stump varies. The stump is measured from the joint line to the distal end of the stump, with the knee flexed to 90°. Prosthetic fitting can be achieved from as little as 7 cm to as long as the musculo-tendonous junction of the calf muscles.

For children, a below-knee amputation does not affect the upper epiphyseal plate of the tibia, and therefore the stump grows with the child, unlike an above-knee stump.

It must be noted that in vascular cases the stump can be slow to heal: patients may have to wait some time before prosthetic re-education can commence and they may become frustrated. The continued use, however, of the early mobility aid and exercises (Chs 4 and 5) helps to maintain the function and mobility of the patient during this slow healing stage.

It is known that 30% of vascular primary amputees lose their second leg within 3 years and if only one of the amputations is a below-knee, function and mobility will be better.

There are, however, a few *contra-indications* to selecting this level of amputation:

a. Hemiplegic patients requiring an amputation on the affected side should never have this level selected, as however minimal the abnormal reflex neurological patterns may appear prior to surgery, a flexor pattern will emerge or increase following surgery, making prosthetic rehabilitation impossible. This type of patient is usually most suited for an above-knee amputation.

b. Any patient assessed as unfit for prosthetic re-education may encounter the following problems with a below-knee stump which may lead to surgical revision at a higher level:
— Muscle imbalance resulting in knee flexion contracture
— Severe damage and tissue breakdown of the stump caused by knocking the furniture while manipulating the wheelchair.

c. The condition of the knee joint prior to surgery must be carefully assessed. A grossly unstable, painful or flexed joint will not control a prosthesis easily. Conditions such as rheumatoid arthritis, osteoarthrosis and ligamentous instability may initially appear stable enough to control this level of amputation, but it must be remembered that these can deteriorate with time. Patients with little range of movement, or an arthrodesed knee, are unlikely to benefit from this level of amputation.

Many other problems, such as wasted muscles in the lower leg, adherent scars, uneven bone contours, skin grafts and poor sensation, can be prosthetically rehabilitated with success at this below-knee level, providing the surgeon is adept and imaginative when fashioning the stump.

THE PATELLAR TENDON BEARING PROSTHESIS

This prosthesis allows the patient to walk with a natural free knee gait from the onset of prosthetic re-education. It is suitable for patients who have a stump in which there is minimal oedema.

Its advantages are that it is easy to apply, easy to use and cosmetically acceptable. The disadvantage is that the fit has to be intimate and this is difficult to achieve in patients whose stump volume fluctuates, e.g. diabetics, patients with chronic cardiac problems and patients taking diuretics.

Maintenance of an intimate fit means that frequent adjustments to the socket may be required. This can be a problem when there are either transport difficulties or the patient lives a long distance from the prosthetist. The patient cannot continue with prosthetic re-education if skin problems are caused by the socket. Alternative means of mobility (e.g. crutches or wheelchair) must be used. This can interrupt the patient's functional independence at home.

Close liaison is required between the physiotherapist and the prosthetist in the early stages of gait re-education with a PTB. There is a wide variety of interchangeable socket designs and suspensions available for the stump with fitting or skin problems. Great skill and imagination are required of both professions to overcome difficulties, and reassurance must be given to the patient that a correct fit may take some time and effort to achieve if the stump is not 'ideal'.

If after many attempts with different varieties of PTB prosthesis success is still elusive, a conventional thigh corset prosthesis may be required in order to relieve the forces on the stump (see p. 144).

Sockets

There is a variety of socket designs, some self-suspending and some requiring additional suspension; however, all are based on the pressure-tolerant

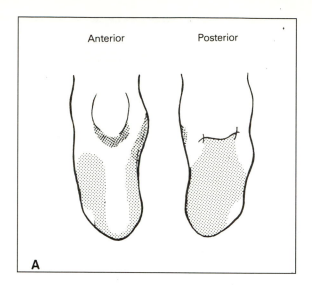

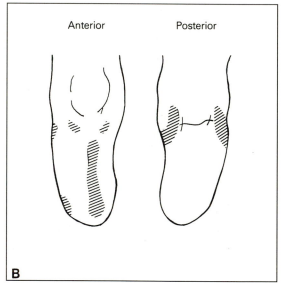

Fig. 13.1   The pressure-tolerant (A) and pressure-sensitive (B) areas of the below-knee stump.

and pressure-sensitive areas of the below-knee stump.

The following weightbearing areas are emphasised (see Fig. 13.1A):

— The patellar tendon area
— The medial flare of the tibia and tibial condyle (and to a lesser extent the lateral flare)
— The posterior muscle bulk.

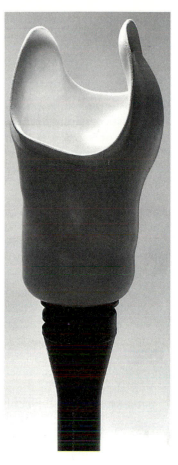

Fig. 13.2 The patella tendon bearing/supracondylar socket. (Photograph by kind permission of C. A. Blatchford & Sons Ltd.)

Weightbearing is relieved in the following areas (Fig. 13.1B):

— The distal end of the tibia
— The crest of the tibia and tibial tubercle
— The head of the fibula
— Hamstring tendon insertions, both medial and lateral.

Patella tendon bearing (PTB) socket

This socket is intimately fitting with minimal relief over the pressure-sensitive areas. There is a patella tendon bar filling the space between the inferior pole of the patella and the tibial tubercle. The socket fits closely under the medial tibial condyle and there is good support to the popliteal surface of the stump and a flare to accommodate the hamstring tendons (see Fig. 13.7).

Patella tendon bearing/supracondylar socket

This socket is basically the same as the PTB socket, but the medial and lateral walls are high enough to enclose the medial and lateral femoral condyles, thus increasing the suspension (see Fig. 13.2).

Prosthèse tibiale supracondylienne (PTS)

This is as the PTB/supracondylar socket, but the anterior wall of the socket is raised to encompass the patella, further increasing the suspension.

The above sockets are made on a plaster cast taken of the stump when the patient is sitting. This negative cast is then made into a positive mould and the prosthetist rectifies the mould by building up the pressure-tolerant areas of the stump and relieving the pressure-sensitive areas. A soft liner is made on this plaster mould and a thermoplastic socket is worn over the liner. The socket is set in a slight degree of flexion and adduction to ensure correct weightbearing, particularly on the patella tendon, which is emphasised by the counterforce of the upper part of the posterior wall.

Köndylen bettung Munster (KBM)

With this socket weight is taken much more on the medial flare of the tibia and the patella tendon bar is not so marked. The casting technique is very different and is done with the patient standing.

Sockets with silicone liners, e.g. Iceross (Icelandic Roll-on Silicone Socket) or 3S (Silicone Suction Socket)

These are made of softer materials and are very useful for neuropathic stumps, heavily skin-grafted stumps and difficult scars. No stump sock is worn and the socket is self-suspending. The soft liner attaches to a hard shell (PTB shape) by either a cord or a ratchet mechanism. Care is needed not to damage the liner with long fingernails or sharp objects. These sockets are expensive and their cost effectiveness is being evaluated.

Suspension

Leather cuff. This passes immediately above the patella, fits snugly around the femoral condyles and fastens firmly posterolaterally, usually with a buckle. Angled side straps attach the cuff to the socket (see Fig. 13.7E, p. 150). The actual design of the supracondylar cuff can vary. Some have an elasticated middle portion, which is particularly useful for patients with ill-defined contours about the knee.

Elastic stocking. The female amputee can suspend the temporary prosthesis with a specially made elastic stocking attached to a suspender belt (see Fig. 13.3).

Pick-up strap added to the cuff suspension and attached to a waist belt may be required if the contour of the patient's knee is ill-defined or the stump is short (see Fig. 13.4).

Elastic sleeve suspension fits over the distal femur and the proximal socket; it may be elastic stocking material, e.g. Juzo suspension sleeve, or Neoprene.

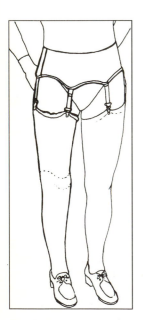

Fig. 13.3 Elastic stocking suspension for the PTB.

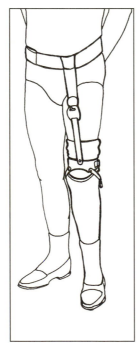

Fig. 13.4 A pick-up strap attached to the supracondylar cuff of the PTB improves suspension.

Patients require strong hands with maximal dexterity to apply these sleeves.

PROSTHESIS WITH THIGH CORSET
(see Fig. 13.5)

This type of prosthesis is indicated when a patient has tried unsuccessfully to tolerate a PTB (of varying designs) or when a patient is accustomed to a thigh corset and does not wish to change.

Examples of conditions which may not suit a PTB are:

— An unstable knee joint. This may be stabilised by the side steels of the conventional thigh corset which act as a caliper.
— A knee flexion contracture of more than 25°.
— A very short stump.
— A hyper- or hyposensitive (possibly anaesthetic) stump, or one with adherent scarring. Skin-grafted stumps may not be tough enough for a PTB.
— Malformation of the patella or knee joint area, e.g. congenital abnormality of the patella, occasionally patellectomy, or deformities caused by fractures.
— A patient whose occupation or hobbies involve heavy work; for example, farming, mountaineering, oil rig workers, etc. may need a conventional thigh corset prosthesis for work, but are often supplied with a PTB for social activities.

Those established wearers who would like to change from a thigh corset to a PTB prosthesis will need to be well motivated, have time to adapt, and be prepared to commit themselves to a muscle strengthening, gait and function retraining programme. This is to be encouraged, as in later life the established below-knee amputee may suffer from peripheral vascular disease and the thigh corset will restrict arterial flow to the stump, causing claudication discomfort.

Thigh corset

This is made of blocked leather with a front fastening and may be ischial or buttock weight-bearing; some weight is taken through the length of the corset itself.

Side steels

These extend either side of the thigh corset down to the lower leg, with uniaxial free knee joints. Very occasionally a locking mechanism may be supplied.

Socket

The below-knee stump is contained in the shank, which is made of either metal, wood, or plastic.

The socket is usually proximal weightbearing and made to fit around the upper half of the stump approximately 3 cm from the lower pole of the patella.

With a metal shank, a blocked leather slip socket is always present (see Fig. 13.6). This leather slip socket is made on a plaster cast taken of the patient's stump. It is placed into the shank in such a way that allows both it and the stump to move

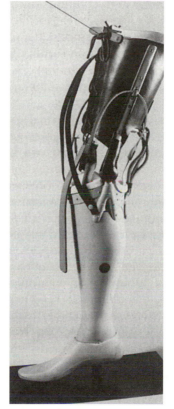

Fig. 13.5 The conventional prosthesis with corset and side steels.

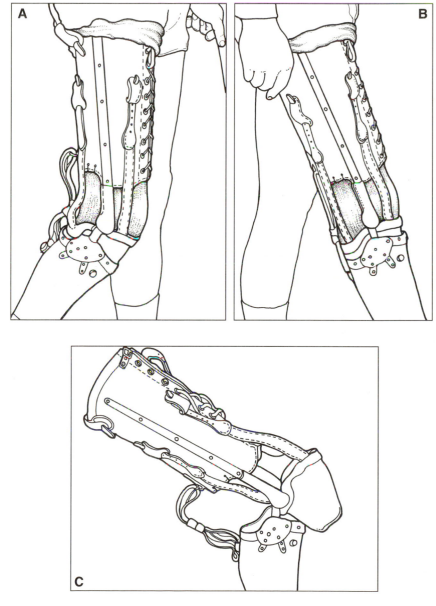

Fig. 13.6 The blocked leather slip socket. (A) and (B) show how it moves with the below-knee stump during walking. (C) shows the slip socket lifted out of the metal shank.

when the patient is sitting, thus protecting the stump from knocking against the shank. Sometimes there are elastic straps from the thigh corset attaching to this slip socket in order to maintain firm contact with the stump while the patient is walking and sitting. This is particularly useful for a very short below-knee stump or where scarring is present.

Backstrap

A leather strap attaches the thigh corset to the shank posteriorly to prevent hyperextension at the knee.

Suspension

This type of prosthesis may be self-suspending, although the following auxiliary suspension may be used:

— A waist belt suspension with one anterior strap extending to below the knee which aids swing through, and one posterior downstrap attaching to the corset.
— A shoulder strap, which crosses over the opposite shoulder from the amputation, and fastens with anterior and posterior straps.
— Very occasionally a rigid pelvic band is used.

CHECK OF THE PTB PROSTHESIS

A full explanation of the correct weightbearing areas must be given to the patient by the physiotherapist. This must be fully comprehended by the patient because the fit of this prosthesis is intimate. It is essential that the skin is checked regularly during the day, *at least every 5 minutes* to begin with; eventually this skin checking will have to become the patient's responsibility. If any redness or soreness is noted the patient must stop walking and remove the prosthesis immediately.

The most satisfactory method of checking the fit of the socket can be achieved when the physiotherapist applies the prosthesis.

Sitting

The patient should be sitting, the affected leg suitably undressed and the stump held in about 40°

flexion at the knee. The *liner of the socket* should be eased over the stump and stump sock; in this way it is possible to feel the correct position, i.e. the weightbearing bar of the socket is in direct contact with the patellar tendon of the patient. The patient's stump should be fully supported by the liner, i.e. there should be total surface bearing with no obvious gaps, either distally or around the rim of the liner and condyles. It may be necessary to fill the distal end of the liner with pieces of cut foam or unravelled wool (e.g. from an old stump sock) to ensure distal tissue support.

The physiotherapist should then apply the *outer hard socket* over the liner in the same way and it should slip into position easily. The fit between the two should be perfect. The patient should then flex the knee to 90° and the physiotherapist should check that there is adequate flaring of the posterior brim to accommodate the hamstring tendons. There should not be excessive bulging of tissue in the popliteal area.

The position of the *supracondylar cuff* suspension should be such that it traps the patella between the cuff and the anterior brim of the socket. It must be firmly fastened but with enough space to allow two fingers to pass underneath it; the tourniquet effect is to be avoided. The patient should be sufficiently dexterous to fasten the cuff correctly. If a buckle is unmanageable or unsightly, Velcro can be used. The physiotherapist should make sure that the side straps are firm when the knee is in extension and a little looser when the knee is flexed. If an elastic stocking is used the patient must be able to manipulate the suspenders. If not, the suspender strap can be fixed with Velcro.

If the *socket is difficult to apply* the following remedies may be tried:

1. The physiotherapist may decrease the number and the thickness of the stump socks. It is possible to use a PTB wearing only a nylon sock, providing a careful check is kept by both physiotherapist and patient. It is often necessary to juggle with socks for several days until the stump has settled down and the oedema reduced.

2. Sometimes the liner fits, but the hard outer socket appears too tight, i.e. it is either very difficult or impossible to ease over the liner. This may occur if the shape of the stump is bulbous distally. If

the physiotherapist puts a nylon stump sock over the liner, the outer socket is much easier to apply with less friction. A pop sock or talcum powder can be used for this if there is no nylon stump sock available.

3. If the stump is grossly oedematous and the prosthesis is impossible to apply it may be possible to reduce the oedema by the following methods:

a. Place the patient supine, with the stump in high elevation and apply a stump bandage correctly or Juzo sock (see Ch. 3). Leave the stump in this position for 1 hour, instructing the patient to perform stump muscle contractions before trying to apply the prosthesis again.

b. If available, a variable air pressure machine (Flowtron, Jobst, etc.) should be used with the stump elevated (see Ch. 3).

4. There may be other reasons for the tightness of the socket and the physiotherapist should always investigate the persistently oedematous stump. If the remaining leg also shows oedema, the patient may have poorly controlled congestive cardiac failure or diabetes. The patient may also have put on weight, and a weight variation of more than 2.5 kg can affect stump volume. A medical opinion may be necessary.

5. If the socket is too loose, the physiotherapist must increase the number and types of stump socks. The maximum number of socks permitted is one cotton and two wool. After this, the physiotherapist must contact the prosthetist as the PE Lite liner may have to be lined or a new socket made.

Standing

The patient then stands supported and partially weightbears through the prosthesis, and a further check of the prosthesis is made. About 0.5 cm of PE Lite liner should be visible above the rim of the socket. The anterior brim of the socket extends to the middle of the patella. The physiotherapist should check that the shoe worn is the one for which the prosthesis was measured and that the patient is wearing a pair of shoes.

If the patient reports discomfort when standing, has reduced sensation in the stump, or is unable to report reliably, the physiotherapist must check that there is sufficient tissue contact between the distal end of the stump and the liner, but not undue pressure. This may be determined by inserting a piece of Blu-Tack or Plasticine inside the liner prior to application of the prosthesis. After the patient has been standing for a few minutes, the prosthesis is removed and the Blu-Tack or Plasticine examined for marks of indentation from the stump sock. 'Touch' pressure for tissue support must be present. If it is not, cut pieces of shaped foam or unravelled wool (e.g. from an old stump sock) should be inserted into the liner to produce this tissue support. This is necessary to prevent terminal oedema and undue stress on a scar line which is often directly over the cut end of the tibia.

However, if the indentations on the Blu-Tack are heavy, the stump has sunk too far into the socket. This usually occurs if the socket is too large, in which case the physiotherapist should:

— Add up to one cotton and two woollen stump socks without losing the shape of the stump, relative to the socket. If more socks are required, a stump sock can be placed between the PE Lite liner and the hard socket.
— Check the cuff and side straps, elastic stocking, or Neoprene sleeve suspension for firmness.
— Check to see if the set of the socket in flexion is sufficient to maintain correct weightbearing on the patellar tendon bar.
— Add a popliteal pad between the liner and the hard socket in order to push the stump forwards on to the patellar tendon bar.

Walking

The patient then walks with the PTB, and a dynamic check of the fit is made. There should be no discomfort in the distal end of the stump and minimal pistoning between the stump and the prosthesis should be present. A line drawn on the stump sock along the posterior brim is a useful guide to check pistoning when the patient is observed from behind. This should be no more than 1 cm. The cuff should maintain adequate suspension throughout the gait cycle.

If excessive pistoning occurs the suspension may not be adequate. The angled side straps may be too loose and require adaptation. A 'pick-up' added to the cuff suspension and attached to a waist belt may be required if the contour of the patient's knee is ill defined, or the stump is short (see Fig. 13.4). If this problem continues, a different shaped socket (e.g. PTS) may need to be tried.

All patients will report discomfort over the correct weightbearing areas during the early stages. It takes time for the skin to harden over these areas and the patient must be reassured. Those patients wearing PTB/supracondylar or PTS sockets may report redness and/or soreness over the femoral condyles and the inferior and lateral borders of the patella. The skill is in developing a balance between an acceptable level or 'new soreness' (as a good suspension of these sockets is dependent on a snug fit) and an actual pressure sore. However, the following measures may be utilised to improve the patient's comfort:

— To reduce friction, a nylon sock may be worn between the patient's skin and stump sock.
— To protect the skin, a small Airstrip can be applied over the patellar tendon. However, this must be removed at night.
— To prevent any skin breakdown occurring, the physiotherapist must constantly check the condition of the skin of the stump. Gait re-education may have to be limited to short periods of time during the initial phases. Open areas are a disaster for the patient, particularly for those with diabetes and marked peripheral vascular disease.

When checking the PTB prosthesis the physiotherapist should be aware that patients with peripheral vascular disease may be experiencing ischaemic pain in the stump. This will not be helped by alterations to the fit of the prosthesis. Ischaemia may be detected by:

— A blue/red mottled stump, cold to the touch, which blanches on elevation
— The reporting of intense pain
— An indolent wound in which slough is present.

It should be realised that further surgery may be required and an appointment with the patient's hospital surgeon must be obtained. A full report from the physiotherapist must be sent to the surgeon.

CHECK OF THE CONVENTIONAL PROSTHESIS WITH THIGH CORSET AND SIDE STEELS

The physiotherapist should check that the patient is not wearing a stump bandage, but the correct stump sock.

Standing

The patient must be standing with the knee fully extended and weight evenly distributed. If the prosthesis is ischial weightbearing, the physiotherapist should carry out the check in exactly the same way as for the above-knee prosthesis (see Ch. 11).

The thigh corset should be fastened correctly. It must not be fastened too tightly as circulation embarrassment can occur. The length of the prosthesis is checked in the same way as for the above-knee prosthesis (see Ch. 11).

The below-knee socket must be correctly positioned so that some weight is taken on the patellar tendon area and upper part of the stump. If this seems too loose, a short below-knee stump sock can be added.

The auxiliary suspension should be firm when the patient stands erect and it should maintain the correct position of the prosthesis throughout the gait cycle.

Sitting

The prosthetic knee joint must be aligned with the patient's knee. If there is a slip socket present, the physiotherapist should check that it moves with the stump when the patient sits down. The buckles on the elastic straps attaching the slip socket to the thigh corset can be adjusted if necessary.

If there is no slip socket present and the patient experiences discomfort in the stump when sitting with the knee flexed to 90°, the physiotherapist should contact the prosthetist and enquire about the possibility of altering the prosthesis.

If discomfort persists when the patient is sitting, the physiotherapist should remove and re-apply the prosthesis to check for correct positioning and fastening of the thigh corset. Patients can 'fasten' themselves either 'in' or 'out' of the prosthesis.

Walking

The blocked leather thigh corset will expand and soften slightly with the patient's body heat; re-fastening of the corset after about an hour of gait re-education may be necessary. However, the patient should not fasten the thigh corset too tightly as this produces the 'tourniquet' effect.

Pistoning can be checked more easily by observation of the patient from behind. After checking the fastening of the thigh corset and auxiliary suspension, and the number and thickness of the stump socks, the physiotherapist may decide that further suspension is required and must contact the prosthetist.

The adductor region must be comfortable. The physiotherapist should check that the prosthesis has been applied at the correct angle, that the stump socks are well pulled up out over the brim of the thigh corset and that the patient is using the hip extensor muscle maximally at heel strike. (If the patient has a flexion contracture at the knee joint it is possible that a hip flexion contracture is also present which may not have been accommodated in the thigh corset.) If further adjustments are needed the physiotherapist should contact the prosthetist.

The physiotherapist should check and if necessary re-educate the patient's knee joint function to prevent hyperextension at heel strike. If this hyperextension persists, the backstrap can be tightened.

The alignment of the prosthesis should be observed throughout the gait cycle and if obvious abnormality is present the physiotherapist should contact the prosthetist for adjustments.

FUNCTIONAL RE-EDUCATION IN THE BELOW-KNEE PROSTHESIS

Application

The PTB prosthesis (see Fig. 13.7)

1. The patient should be sitting down, the amputated side undressed apart from underwear.
2. The stump sock should be pulled up smoothly over the stump. If more than one stump sock is used, they must be applied separately (Fig. 13.7A).
3. The PE Lite liner should be eased onto the stump with the knee held in about 40° flexion (Fig. 13.7B & C).
4. The supracondylar cuff should be folded forward over the anterior aspect of the hard socket before the prosthesis is applied over the liner. The hard socket is pulled on, with the knee in flexion. It may be necessary to exert downward pressure through the stump, by pressing the heel of the prosthesis onto the floor, in order to slide the stump right down into the socket (Fig. 13.7D).
5. The cuff is pulled up over the knee and must be fastened securely (Fig. 13.7E).
6. The stump sock should be pulled up firmly. (Some patients fold the sock back down over the cuff.)
7. If elastic stocking suspension is used, the patient must be able to stand to fasten the posterior suspender (see Fig. 13.8). Similarly, if an elasticated cuff or Neopren sleeve is used, they should be applied while standing.

The PTB/supracondylar and PTS sockets. The patient should slide the stump into these sockets by 'climbing in' over the posterior brim so that the stump is not caught by the supracondylar flares. The knee joint can be in near extension and the socket should be at a forward-tilted angle of 45° to the stump.

The KBM socket. The patient is standing. The stump sock is applied, then a tubular stocking is put over sock and stump. The patient then draws the stump down into the liner by pulling the tubular stocking out through an opening in the liner. The stocking is then folded back over the liner and the hard shell outer socket is applied.

The prosthetist will be the person determining the exact method of application of this socket and it is essential that the physiotherapist is aware of this and is in communication.

NB: This pull-in technique can be used to draw a fleshy stump into any PTB-type liner, if it is a tight fit. Care should be taken not to pinch the tissues in the split made in the liner to accommodate the large circumference being pulled through it.

Removal

1. The patient should sit down.
2. The suspension should be undone.

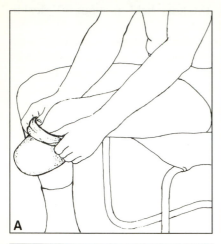

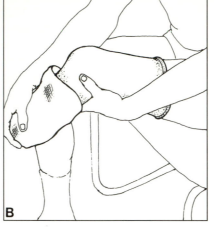

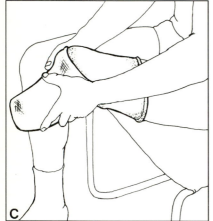

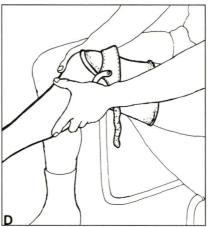

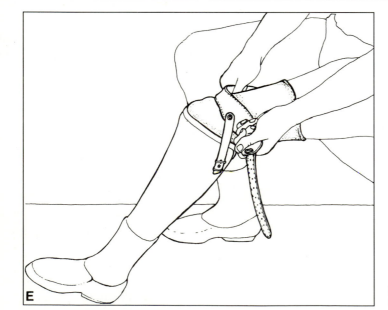

Fig. 13.7 Application of the PTB prosthesis.

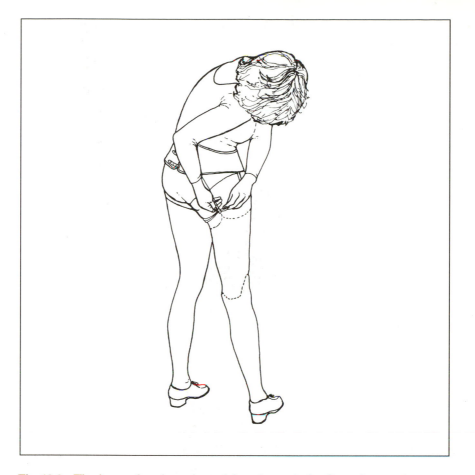

Fig. 13.8 The degree of trunk rotation and dexterity required to fasten the posterior suspender with elastic stocking suspension for the PTB.

3. With the patient's knee held in 30–40° flexion, the stump should be eased out of the prosthesis. Usually the socket, liner and sock all come off together.
4. The skin of the stump should be inspected. The correct weightbearing areas may be red; this is normal. However, the weight-relieved areas should not be red or rubbed. Alterations to the prosthesis may be necessary if this persists. No terminal oedema of the stump should be present.

Dressing

If a skirt is worn, there will be no difficulty in applying this prosthesis either before or after dressing. If tight trousers or jeans are worn it is better to dress the PTB before applying it to the stump.

In the early stages of gait re-education, when frequent examination of the skin of the stump has to be made, it is better if tight trousers are not worn, as it is very difficult to slip the prosthesis on and off. Shorts are more suitable at this stage.

The conventional thigh corset prosthesis

This is difficult to apply. The patient must sit down in order to ease on the prosthesis, but then must be able to stand up to put downward pressure on the prosthesis before fastening the corset. Considerable dexterity and balance are required. The auxiliary suspension must be fastened while the patient is sitting, but adjusted when the patient is standing, to ensure a firm fit.

If the patient is unable to manage the lacing of the thigh corset it can be changed to straps and buckles, or Velcro. This is particularly important for diabetics, who may have diminished sensation in the fingers and visual impairment.

GAIT RE-EDUCATION

The PTB prosthesis

The main consideration that the physiotherapist has to take into account here is that the length of time that the patient can spend wearing the PTB during gait re-education is limited initially. This is because the tolerance of the skin over the weight-bearing areas of the stump can only be increased very gradually.

It is the physiotherapist's responsibility to constantly check the stump and decide when activity must be interrupted for an interval to allow the skin to recover. Frequently, patients who are enthusiastic wish to continue for too long and must be persuaded to rest. As a general guide, gait re-education initially should not be longer than 1 hour morning and afternoon. It must be made clear to the patient that walking is not permitted at home until skin tolerance to the weightbearing areas is satisfactory and independence has been achieved with a suitable walking aid in the physiotherapy department.

The aim of gait re-education with the PTB is to achieve a normal gait pattern, and it should start in the parallel bars. Most of these patients will have used an early mobility aid before the delivery of their PTB and will be accustomed to hip hitching and walking with a stiff knee. A smooth hip and knee flexion prior to toe off must be taught. At heel strike, controlled knee flexion is required in order to prevent either hyper-extension or sudden knee flexion. Sometimes a different type of shoe with a softer heel is needed to assist this controlled knee flexion action.

Even stride length and rhythm should be encouraged. A mirror and video are very helpful visual aids for the patient. The physiotherapist must observe the gait pattern from in front, at the sides and behind.

When a near normal gait pattern has been achieved in the parallel bars, the patient then progresses to using walking aids. Although the majority of PTB users progress to walking sticks very quickly, the elderly and frail may need the full support and confidence given by a walking frame.

In the early stages it may not be possible to use the normal gait pattern on stairs or ramps, but as knee control and muscle strength improve, the patient's ability to manage these obstacles increases. Later on, all PTB wearers can climb stairs normally, with the exception of the elderly and frail.

There are no special methods for getting up after a fall. However, before getting up it is important that the patient remains seated on the floor for a short time to overcome shock and gather walking aids.

Those patients who progress from the locked knee above-knee/below-knee temporary prosthesis to a free knee prosthesis (either PTB or conventional thigh corset type) should always return initially to the parallel bars.

Thigh corset prosthesis

Patients using a thigh corset prosthesis will tend to control the prosthesis using hip muscles more than knee muscles. This produces a rather uneven gait with an energetic swing phase and pronounced heel strike. The thigh muscles will, in time, atrophy through disuse.

Because of the different type of muscle control used with each prosthesis, it may be difficult to convert an experienced conventional thigh corset prosthesis wearer to a PTB wearer.

PROTHESES INFORMATION

Detailed information regarding prostheses available in the UK can be obtained from the manufacturers. The addresses are listed in the Appendix.

REFERENCES

Boldingh E J K, Van Pijkeren T, Wijkmans D W 1985 A study on the value of the modified KBM prothesis compared with other types of prosthesis. Prosthetics and Orthotics International 9: 79–82

Donn J M, Porter D, Roberts V C 1989 The effect of footwear mass on gait patterns of unilateral below-knee emputees. Prosthetics and Orthotics International 10: 139–141

Enoka R M, Miller D I, Burgess E M 1982 Below-knee amputee running gait. American Journal of Physical Medicine 61 (2): 66–84

Fleurant F W, Alexander J 1980 Below knee amputation and rehabilitation of amputees. Surgery, Gynaecology and Obstetrics 151: 41–44

Isakov E, Mizrahi J, Susak Z, Onna I 1992 A Swedish knee cage for stabilising short below-knee stumps. Prosthetics and Orthotics International 16: 114–117

Kegel B, Burgess E M, Starr T W, Daly W K 1981 Effects of isometric muscle training on residual limb volume, strength, and gait of below-knee amputees. Physical Therapy 61 (10): 1419–1426

Renstrom P, Grinby G, Larsson E 1983 Thigh muscle strength in below-knee amputees. Scandinavian Journal of Rehabilitation 9: 163–173

Robinson K P 1972 Long-posterior-flap myoplastic below-knee amputation in ischaemic disease. Lancet Jan 22: 193–195

Robinson K P, Hoile R, Coddington T 1982 Skew flap myoplastic below-knee amputation: a preliminary report. British Journal of Surgery 69 (9): 554–557

Saadah E S M 1988. Bilateral below-knee amputee 107 years old and still wearing artificial limbs. Prosthetics and Orthotics International 12: 105–106

Vittas D, Larsen T K, Jansen E C 1986. Body sway in below-knee amputees. Prosthetics and Orthotics International 10: 139–141

Weiss J, Middleton L, Gonzalez E, Lovelace R E 1983 The thigh corset: its effect on the quadriceps muscle and its role in prosthetic suspension. Orthotics and Prosthetics 37 (3): 58–62

Wilson A B 1979 Lightweight prostheses. Prosthetics and Orthotics International 3: 150–151

Wirta R W et al 1990 Analysis of below-knee suspension systems: effect on gait. Journal of Rehabilitation Research and Development 27(4): 385–396

14. The Symes and partial foot levels of amputation

THE SYMES AMPUTATION

This was first performed by James Syme of Edinburgh in 1842. The amputation is a disarticulation of the ankle: the os calcis is removed and the tibia is sectioned just proximal to its distal articular surface, with the removal of the medial malleolus. The lateral malleolus is removed at the same level. The heel pad and tough skin overlying it are retained and swung forward to cover the ends of the tibia and fibula. The suture line is anterior. It is essential postoperatively that the dressings maintain the heel pad in position, so that a firm contact is established between it and the bone ends. The heel pad should not slip posteriorly. A frequent cause of failure of this level of amputation is related to the position, fixation or viability of the heel pad. The ideal stump should be capable of total endbearing, with or without a prosthesis, and should be short enough to allow a prosthetic foot to be fitted to a normal shoe, i.e. there should be a ground clearance of the stump of at least 4 cm. If the stump cannot fully endbear, a PTB brim is needed to the proximal socket.

This stump has similar attributes to those of knee disarticulation, i.e. it is a long endbearing stump, with proprioceptive properties. The indications for this procedure are:

1. Trauma
2. Congenital shortening of the leg
3. Chronic infection of the foot.

Trauma

Severe trauma to the forefoot, provided that the plantar heel pad is intact, can be treated with this level of amputation. Cold trauma, i.e. frostbite, is another reason for this amputation.

Congenital shortening of the leg

The foot may be normal in appearance but useless functionally in this situation. Prosthetic management with extension prostheses (see Ch. 2) can be facilitated by removal of the foot.

Chronic infections of the foot

Patients with perforating ulcers, possibly diabetic in origin, or infections secondary to a neuropathy (diabetes, leprosy and spina bifida) may benefit from this level of amputation, providing there is adequate sensation in the heel pad. In countries where sophisticated drugs are less readily available, this level of amputation may be the first choice of treatment for these conditions.

Very occasionally, this level may be selected where there is distal diabetic vascular disease, but it is rarely successful in atherosclerosis.

THE SYMES PROSTHESIS

The patient can mobilise very early, after the wound has healed, in a prosthesis. The materials used for the construction of the socket are blocked leather and thermoplastics.

The enclosed metal Symes prosthesis

This prosthesis is cosmetically acceptable and many women with this level of amputation favour it. There is a leather socket, with a posterior flap opening which fits inside the metal shin and attaches to it. The foot is uniaxial or low profile SACH.

The all plastic Symes prosthesis
(see Figs 14.1 and 14.2)

This prosthesis has improved cosmesis, with a smooth outline and reduced ankle width. There is a Pelite liner which fits into the hard plastic outer socket. There is no access panel and it is described as a 'push fit'. This is similar to the through-knee plastic socket (see Ch. 12). However, the Canadian window type Symes prosthesis has a posterior or medial access panel held in place by Velcro straps or elastic cuffs. The foot is as for the enclosed metal Symes with the addition of the Quantum foot.

CHECK OF THE SYMES PROSTHESIS

The physiotherapist should check that the weight-bearing areas of the stump for which the prosthesis is constructed are being utilised correctly.

The total endbearing prosthesis

As stated previously, some stumps can be totally endbearing and some stumps have to have the weight distributed proximally. The heel pad should not become red or sore during walking. The scar line must be watched carefully during the early stages of prosthetic use.

Patients who have a hyposensitive stump should have gait re-education limited to 1 hour morning and afternoon. The physiotherapist must frequently remove the prosthesis and examine the stump for areas of redness, rubbing or spots. The patient must be taught to examine the stump, using a mirror to check the heel pad. If a totally endbearing prosthesis is used and the patient complains of discomfort on the heel pad, the reasons may be that:

— The stump sock has not been pulled up over the stump correctly and has possibly formed wrinkles over the weightbearing areas.
— A different type of stump sock may be needed, e.g. the thick terry-cotton sock.

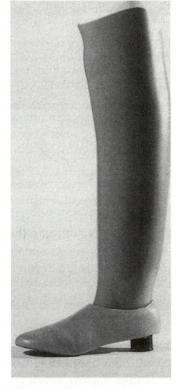

Fig. 14.1 The all plastic Symes prosthesis.

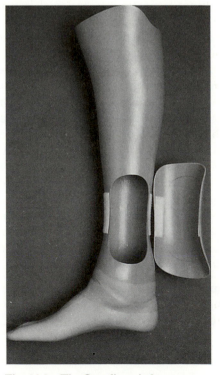

Fig. 14.2 The Canadian window-type Symes prosthesis. (Photograph from Redhead et al.)

— The socket is too loose, which thus allows excessive movement of the stump to take place.
— The socket is too tight, causing constriction of circulation.
— The socket is ill-fitting around the bony contours of the stump.
— The set of the prosthetic foot may need adjustment in order to prevent excessive shear forces, particularly at heel strike and toe off.

The physiotherapist can alter the end pad with pieces of foam, change the type and thickness of the stump sock and check that the prosthesis has been correctly applied.

The partial endbearing prosthesis

Some patients need to distribute the weight between the following areas: the distal end of the stump, the length of the stump, the medial tibial condyle and the patellar tendon. However, some are totally proximally weighbearing.

Prosthetic re-education in the early stages must be limited to short sessions to allow for progressive hardening of the skin over the proximal weight-bearing areas (see Ch. 13).

It must be remembered that if the physiotherapist is unable to solve a fitting problem the prosthetist must be contacted for further alterations to be made.

The position of the heel pad over the bone ends can slip after a period of prosthetic use. Discomfort will be reported in this area and no amount of alteration to the prosthesis will help. The hospital surgeon must be contacted with a view to revision of the stump.

PARTIAL FOOT AMPUTATION

The mid tarsal amputation (Chopart)

The is a disarticulation between the talus and calcaneus proximally and the navicular and cuboid distally.

The tarsometatarsal amputation (Lisfranc)

This is a disarticulation of the forefoot at the tarsometatarsal line.

These amputations are rarely carried out, the only indications being severe crush injury of the forefoot and frostbite. Occasionally they are carried out for infection of the forefoot. The disadvantages of these levels of amputation are that the stump tends to be pulled into equinus by the unbalanced pull of the Achilles tendon and into inversion by tibialis anterior. Also, even after the wound has healed, the skin which remains over the antero-inferior aspect of the stump tends to develop callosities and corns with prosthetic wear. These can become painful and troublesome.

Physiotherapy is required pre-operatively and immediately postoperatively in order to maintain ankle joint mobility and the length of the Achilles tendon, thus avoiding the equinus deformity.

Temporary prosthesis

It is unusual to have a temporary prosthesis for this level of amputation because of the slow healing. However, should this be indicated, the physiotherapist, occupational therapist, chiropodist or orthotist can make a temporary weightbearing bootee using thermoplastic material.

The physiotherapist should check the skin of the stump and instruct the patient to examine the stump during the early stages of walking training.

Definitive prosthesis

There are several prostheses for this level of amputation, three of which are described here.

1. A short leather ankle corset attached to a wooden foot which may be worn inside a normal shoe. The patient takes weight through the heel pad and the corset must be securely fastened to prevent a sliding movement of the stump. Full ankle range is maintained.

2. A custom-made silicone socket/slipper is a very cosmetically acceptable alternative (see Fig. 14.3). The advantage of this type is that they may be worn with or without a shoe. The disadvantages are that they are rather sweaty, heavy and the forefoot lever may be insufficiently rigid.

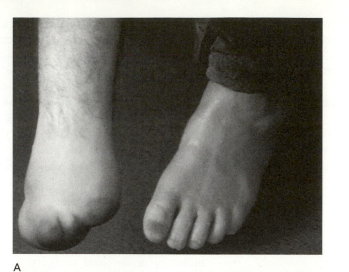

A

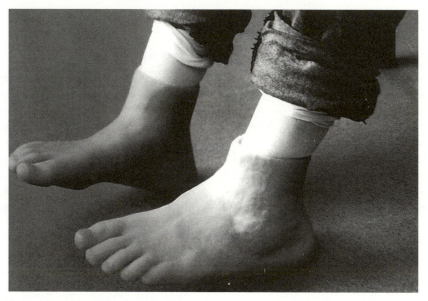

B

Fig. 14.3   A bilateral foot amputee. (A) shows the extent of amputation, (B) shows the cosmetic silicone partial foot prostheses. (Photographs by kind permission of Hugh Steeper Ltd.)

However, this design is very popular with partial foot amputees. Care must be taken when applying silicone feet as the material can be torn.

3. A simple shoe filler made of leather-covered Ortholene, which fits inside a normal shoe.

It should be noted that the design of the prostheses for the Chopart and Lisfranc amputations will be dictated by the weightbearing properties and shape of the individual stumps.

FUNCTIONAL RE-EDUCATION OF THE SYMES AND PARTIAL FOOT LEVELS OF AMPUTATION

Application of the prosthesis

The Symes and most Chopart levels have a stump sock which must be pulled up smoothly to ensure that there are no wrinkles over the weightbearing areas.

With partial foot prostheses, an ordinary but smaller-size wool ankle sock can be worn. Women can wear a cotton slip-on sock. No specific instruction is required for the application of these prostheses.

All partial foot amputees will need to obtain shoes which fit over the prosthesis and some effort may be required in finding a suitable pair.

Gait re-education

Patients with these distal levels of amputation often experience a greater sense of functional loss than those with more proximal levels of amputation.

Balance training is the most important consideration, particularly for the forefoot and first toe amputees. Initially, rhythmic stabilisation in standing and a wobble board can be used, and the physiotherapist must encourage the patient to walk outside over different surfaces such as gravel, rough ground, hills, etc. It is on these surfaces particularly that patients will notice their altered balance reactions.

Loss of push-off is progressively more noticeable the more distal the amputation. Seemingly minor amputations may produce a very uneven gait pattern.

Although one of the benefits of the Symes and Chopart levels is that they are endbearing, enabling the patient to walk without wearing is prosthesis, it should be realised that as the initial cause of amputation is often neuropathic, sensation of the stump is diminished. Therefore, damage may occur which may not be perceived immediately when the patient walks about the home without the prosthesis. If an open area then occurs and becomes infected, re-amputation may be necessary. The physiotherapist should test the sensation of the stump in all distal levels. The danger of damage and the simple measures which can be taken to avoid this must be fully explained to the patient. A home visit is necessary to check out the floor coverings, the presence of loose carpet, tacks, etc. The patient should also be advised to wear a Plastazote bootee as a household slipper, which is made before discharge from hospital.

TRANSMETATARSAL AND TOE AMPUTATIONS

The transmetatarsal level is amputation of the toes proximal to the metatarsal heads. The indications are:

— Trauma.
— Slowly progressive localised gangrene precipitated by minor injury. A high proportion of these patients are diabetic.
— After major reconstruction of large vessels for peripheral vascular disease, the distal part of the foot may not be revascularised and may require amputation.
— Deformity.

Amputation of all the toes is indicated either for extensive trauma or multiple deformities, e.g. rheumatoid arthritis.

Amputation of an individual toe with its corresponding metatarsal is called a 'ray' amputation.

Wherever amputation of the toes is thought to be indicated, due consideration must be given to the stability, biomechanics and viability of the remaining foot. For example, if the first ray is amputated (the most stable ray), weight is then transferred onto the lateral border of the foot which frequently ulcerates and breaks down, particularly if toes four and five are in a poor state. However, if the second ray is removed, a stable situation exists and the foot is more likely to survive.

The full biomechanical assessment that can be made by a chiropodist/podiatrist using force platforms is advisable with these levels of amputation.

Prostheses for distal amputations

Physiotherapists are often asked to make insoles and/or shoes for these patients. This is possible using thermoplastic materials, or alternatively by adapting the patient's own shoes as a temporary measure. It must be remembered, when making these shoes, that sufficient depth should be allowed in order to accommodate the increased depth of the foot and allow sufficient room for extra cushioning needed for the redistribution of weight.

The hospital appliance department and the chiropody service are able to make more permanent and suitable footwear. Custom-made insoles or toe blocks can be made by them and advice given regarding firms which make shoes to measure. In the case of the first toe amputation, an insole with a toe block is needed to prevent friction over the first metatarsal head as this ulcerates easily. For amputation of individual toes a single toe block is required to prevent further distortion of foot shape. This can be made of silicone rubber.

PROSTHESES INFORMATION

Detailed information regarding prostheses available in the UK can be obtained from the manufacturers. The addresses are listed in the Appendix.

REFERENCES

Anderson L, Westin G W, Oppenheim W L 1984 Syme amputation in children: indications, results and long-term follow-up. Journal of Pediatric Orthopaedics 4: 550–554

Bahler A 1986 The biomechanics of the foot. Clinical Prosthetics and Orthotics 10(1): 8–14

Baker W H, Barnes R W 1977 Minor forefoot amputation in patients with low ankle pressure. American Journal of Surgery 133: 331–332

Hayhurst D J 1978 Prosthetic management of a partial-foot amputee. Inter Clinic Information Bulletin 17(1): 11–15

Lange T A, Nasca R J 1984 Traumatic partial foot amputation. Clinical Orthopaedics 185: 137–141

Millstein S G, McCowan S A, Hunter G A 1988 Traumatic partial foot amputations in adults: a long-term review. Journal of Bone and Joint Surgery 70B: 251–254

Mustapha N M, McCard F, Brand A T 1980 Case note — a combined end-bearing and patellar-tendon-bearing prosthesis for Chopart's amputation. Prosthetics and Orthotics International 4(3): 156–158

Oppenheim W L 1991 Fibular deficiency and the indications for Syme's amputation. Prosthetics and Orthotics International 15: 131–136

Pearl M, Johnson R J 1983 An air-ventilated Syme's leg prosthesis. Inter Clinic Information Bulletin 18(5): 5–6

Rubin G 1984 The partial foot amputation. Journal of the American Podiatry Association 74(10): 518–522

Sarmiento A 1972 A modified surgical-prosthetic approach to the Syme's amputation. Clinical Orthopaedics June 85: 11–15

Wagner F W Jr 1977 Amputation of the foot and ankle — current status. Clinical Orthopaedics 122: 62

15. Advanced function

Most patients are discharged from the physiotherapy department as soon as they are walking adequately; however, a fuller lifestyle depends on far more than this. In order to increase amputees' functional capabilities a link should always be maintained between amputees and a physiotherapy department, the community physiotherapy service or the physiotherapist and prosthetist at the DSC.

It should also be remembered that the psychological aspect of picking up the pieces of life again will take differing amounts of time for each individual, and the physiotherapist's approach to increasing activity should be very sensitive. Actually going out of the house for the first time can be daunting, and participation in other activities or sport is only possible when the individual feels confident in himself and his own abilities.

Participation in sports has given many disabled people a new sense of achievement in recent years and there are now many more facilities available. The amputee is able to enjoy a very wide range of activities. Taking part in some form of regular leisure activity provides important social contact and the thrill of competition. The challenge of sport may be the only personal challenge experienced by some individuals, particularly in these days of increased unemployment.

INCREASED FUNCTIONAL ABILITIES

The amputee should already have practised negotiating kerbs, ramps and rough ground, usually in the controlled situation on the physiotherapy department or in a very quiet street.

However, coping in a busy street with bustling pedestrians, uneven pavements, irregular-height kerbs and gutters with a steep camber, requires greater concentration. Crossing a road can be hazardous: it requires forethought, mobility and speed. Drivers may be unaware that the amputee requires more time. Even if the amputee is young and mobile it is advisable, when outside, to carry a walking stick so that the general public are aware of disability requiring consideration.

It may be necessary for above- and through-knee amputees to learn to move quickly for a very short distance to avoid cars and other fast moving hazards. Obviously normal running is impossible but the following method should be used for speed: a stride is taken with the prosthesis; this is followed by a stride, then a hop on the sound leg; this double stance phase allows sufficient time for the prosthesis to swing through and land in full extension; a stride is taken again with the prosthesis (step - step - hop - step). It is best for the patient to attempt this first by holding onto one parallel bar. Then the physiotherapist should practise this with the patient around the gym area of the department.

Amputees who live in a hilly area require special help from the physiotherapist. Descending a steep incline is difficult and unnerving, and the amputee must practise this often by walking sideways with frequent changes of direction. Also, wet leaves, muddy surfaces, high winds and icy conditions are all hazards, and the amputee must be constantly aware of these potential dangers. Suitable footwear can assist balance, and a variety of ferrules are available to stabilise the walking aid.

Escalators present a problem to most amputees (see Fig. 4.17). They should be advised to step both on and off leading with the unaffected leg and keeping a free hand to hold the handrail.

Stepping off an escalator is more difficult as the momentum gained tends to push the trunk forward too fast for the legs. A helper should be in front to clear a space so that the amputee can step on and off with safety.

TRANSPORT

Car

The physiotherapist should be aware of the legal requirements for the vehicle licensing authority to be notified of any changes is a person's medical condition. If amputees are able to drive without having a car adapted, they often do not realise that they are driving illegally if they have not contacted the licensing authority.

All amputees should have been shown how to transfer in and out of a car before discharge from their initial rehabilitation programme. Those who would like to drive must consider certain factors before attempting to drive their own car, or purchasing a new one. Some large driving instruction schools have a 're-learning' programme for those with physical disabilities. At the Mobility Advice and Vehicle Information Units, assessment and advice can be obtained from Department of Transport experts and from specialist therapists. Information concerning these units is available from the local DSC. The physiotherapist should advise even the experienced driver to use one of these re-learning programmes, or to begin driving again as if a novice, and explain that, after a period of hospitalisation, speed of reaction is slowed and the amputee's proprioception is altered.

There are various motoring organisations who can supply more details concerning the law, car adaptations, etc. to the amputee (see Appendix).

Bicycle

Those amputees who were regular cyclists will need to practise on a static bike in the physiotherapy department in order to evaluate whether the prosthesis permits active use of the pedals, and to check mounting and dismounting procedures.

Motorcycle

The choice of model used will depend on the side of the kick-starting mechanism, or the presence of an electric starter, and on the height and location of the pedals, as knee flexion has to be greater than 90°. The amputee must first practise off public roads to achieve proficiency in manoeuvring the machine.

Train and bus

In order to cope with these forms of transport the amputee needs quick, long strides, either up steps or across gaps. To gain confidence, the amputee will often prefer to practise at a quiet time of day with a physiotherapist, before trying it alone or with a friend or relative. If the amputee has a certain route which must be travelled in the rush hour, advice is given to practise the route first at a quiet time of day.

Aeroplane

The majority of amputees must plan the air journey well in advance to check access to the plane and to the lavatories and the leg room available. Even if the amputee is quite mobile it is advisable to ask the airline for a wheelchair to be provided, as airport corridors can be very long. Because of changes in air pressure in the cabin, stump volume may alter, causing fitting difficulties with the prosthesis.

Boats

Travel by sea must also be pre-planned. Wet deck surfaces can be dangerous and the amputee must have good balance to cope with the swell. Stairways can be steep and the location of seats should be ascertained in advance.

SPORT

Actually participating in sport, where the amputee may have to undress or change shoes, will initially make them feel extremely self-conscious and embarrassed; these feelings must be understood, if not overcome, before amputees can move forward into more fulfilling pursuits. Speaking to another amputee who understands these fears and anxieties is often helpful and self-help organisations such as NALD and BASA can provide this support, as well as the professional support available from the members of the treatment team at the local DSC.

The physiotherapist can suggest sport and leisure activities, but must give realistic advice and understand the limitations involved. Young amputees, in particular, are anxious to know, often very soon postoperatively, what their capabilities will be regarding their favourite sport. It will take some time before this advanced function can be achieved possibly as much as 1 year following the amputation. (see Appendix for addresses where advice can be sought).

The main physical considerations before starting a sporting activity are:

— A well-healed and toughened stump
— General muscle strength
— Good stamina.

These are the same considerations as for any individual who is considering starting a sport, and the same training rules apply:

— The technique of the sport must be properly learned
— A correct training programme must be followed
— The amputee must have adequate supervision in the early stages.

If the amputee was proficient at a certain sport before the amputation, it may be easier to return to that same sport rather than learn a new activity. However, returning to such an activity can be very distressing for some people as they are unable to achieve the same level of performance, and it is frustrating to have to compromise their personal standards. Sometimes finding a new challenge is more effective.

For those who were not active in sports prior to amputation, but who would like to have a go, the physiotherapist can advise suitable sports and organisations who can give specific help. The British Sports Association for the Disabled and the British Amputee Sports Association are very good starting points as they have facilities nationally. However, the limited competition here may be too restricting for some individuals and they may wish to join local sports and leisure centres or clubs. The physiotherapist or prosthetist may be able to introduce one amputee to another who is interested in a sport and can often give the

initial help, practical advice and psychological support needed.

It is important that the patients themselves are determined to try and participate, because then they will find a way of succeeding, providing it is within their capabilities. Sport is to be enjoyed: amputees should not be pressurised by others into trying even if they were actively involved prior to amputation. There is a period of psychological adaptation to their condition which must not be rushed and some individuals take longer than others.

The young and fit amputees using prostheses who enjoy sports may require special adaptations, but these must be discussed with the rehabilitation doctor and prosthetist. It may be necessary to fabricate a prosthesis for the special individual requirements of the amputee and the sport.

The following lists contain examples of possible sporting activities available to amputees; they are not comprehensive.

Sports for the less active individual, the elderly and more sedentary

Darts. This can be enjoyed by the amputee either seated or standing, and supported by one walking aid if necessary.

Bowls. Indoors or outdoors; either from a wheelchair or using a prosthesis. The amputee must be able to bend down to the ground (see Fig. 15.1).

Fishing. Access and toilet facilities must be considered. It can be enjoyed both from a wheelchair or seated, or standing.

Billiards, snooker, pool. These slow precision games require only enough balance by the amputee to manage while leaning on the table, but there should be good upper trunk mobility.

Table tennis. Fast reactions are required, but it may be enjoyed from a wheelchair.

Archery. This can be performed from a wheelchair but requires a strong trunk and arms.

Sport for the more active amputee irrespective of age

Swimming. Access to the pool or the sea and availability of helpers must be considered. A lot of advice and direction is needed about getting from the changing room to the pool and vice versa. Local councils have lists of pools that hold special swimming groups for disabled swimmers where help is available for those who feel they need it. (Fig. 15.2).

Croquet. The amputee must be able to balance and walk short distances without a walking aid.

Horse riding. There is a possibility here of discomfort between the stump and socket, particularly for the above-knee amputee who may be more comfortable using a Western-type saddle rather than an English one (Fig.15.3).

Bicycling. Again the saddle is important: a leather touring design is more comfortable. Toe clips should not be used as they can be dangerous if the amputee falls off. A good gripping material on the sole of the shoe will ensure a good hold on the pedals, e.g. good quality sports shoes (Fig. 15.4).

Sailing. The skills required include launching the boat, carrying and loading the equipment, and getting on and off, often from steep, slippery and rocky banks. Therefore most amputees will require a prosthesis with a waterproof latex covering. Some sailing associations have facilities for those in wheelchairs who must have ablebodied helpers present.

Golf. All amputees can enjoy golf, irrespective of the level of amputation. A motorised golf 'buggy' can be used for those with limited walking distance (Fig. 15.5).

Dancing. Disco, ballroom, old time: this can be enjoyed by all, and leaning on one's partner is acceptable!

Shooting. Clay-pigeon shooting is suitable for those who cannot walk far, but excellent standing balance with rotation is required. Rough-shooting is for the more active walker but a peg leg may be more useful for mobility in the undergrowth.

Sports for the very active, vigorous and determined amputee

Skiing. Amputees with above-knee and throughknee levels should start learning without wearing their prosthesis. There are special poles with elbow-crutch tops and outrigger bases to aid balance (Fig. 15.6). Good skiers at these levels can use their prosthesis once basic skills have been mastered, but it does slow them down. A stabilised knee must be set to lock only on very forceful impact. Amputees with below-knee and Symes levels should wear their prosthesis to learn the sport. Very good skiers can achieve higher speeds and skills on one leg. It can be useful to attempt this sport first on a dry slope (Fig. 15.7). One of the major problems for those not wearing their prosthesis is access to the slope, lift and snack bar on one leg. Hopping in a ski boot is almost impossible.

Protection for the stump is vital if a prosthesis is not worn, as injury from cold or trauma must be avoided.

Tobogganing and other snow sports which do not put as much strain on the stump are also possible.

Water skiing. Learning this sport should be attempted on one leg without prosthesis (Fig. 15.8). The below-knee amputee who wishes to use a prosthesis requires a special waterproof design with an extra grip material on the sole. For those on mono-skis, rising up out of the water should be achieved on the unaffected leg and the prosthesis slotted into place when upright. For those wishing to use two skis, rising up from the crouch position may be limited by dorsiflexion of the prosthetic ankle. Is is possible for bilateral amputees to enjoy this sport (Fig. 15.9).

Wind surfing. A non-slip sole on the prosthesis is essential as it is difficult to maintain control on one leg. The above-knee and through-knee amputees require a special peg leg; the below-knee amputee requires a 'beach activity leg'.

Surfing. Most amputees do not use a prosthesis but the below-knee amputee can manage with a 'beach activity leg'. Prone lying or kneeling positions on the board achieve the best balance.

Scuba diving. A 'fin-leg' may be specially made, but many manage without a prosthesis (Fig 15.10).

All those participating in watersport activities using a prosthesis must have full waterproof or specialised materials, and stable suspension (a PTB may need a short thigh corset). A flotation buoy must be attached to the prosthesis, so that it does not sink and is able to be retrieved should it fall off the amputee.

Initially, it is advisable for all amputees who wish to try water sports wearing special prostheses to practise walking, wading, floating and swimming in a shallow guarded swimming pool. This is to test buoyancy and balance.

Hang gliding and parachuting. Highly dangerous for anyone!

Climbing. A prosthesis with very secure suspension should be used.

Hiking and fell walking. Footwear must be suitable. The prosthesis must be very comfortable and well fitting. Extra stump socks should be carried so that changes can be made when necessary. This activity is not for the amputee liable to claudication.

Motorcycle scrambling. Much practice is needed to achieve the correct balance.

Squash, volleyball, badminton, tennis. Although amputees must be agile to attempt these sports, they learn to adapt their game to reduce the need to run about too much. Skilled placing of shots enables them to be competitive (Fig. 15.11).

Running. This is one activity which will show the greatest difference between the above- and below-knee levels. The below-knee amputee can run normally, albeit slower. The above-knee and through-knee amputee have a markedly abnormal running gait, similar to step-hop-step described on page 161. This gait is much slower, appears ungainly and many will not participate in track and field sports because of this. However, there are prosthetic components available which permit a normal running pattern and some young and fit amputees can succeed in this (see Fig. 15.12).

SPECIALISED PROSTHETIC COMPONENTS

The established amputee who has achieved full independence on the first prosthesis may require the next prosthesis to be fitted with specialised components to enable even more active mobility. The components supplied will vary with the individual needs demonstrated by the amputee, with regard to either work, sport or leisure activities.

The availability of specialised components should first be discussed between the amputee and the prosthetist. However, some amputees, once they have become interested in a certain activity, will find out about those components which may help mobility for that activity from a fellow amputee. The amputee must then write to the DSC doctor stating the case for a specialised order.

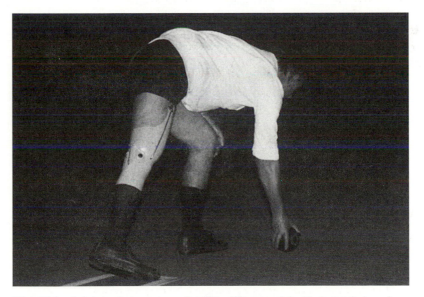

Fig. 15.1   An above-knee amputee bowling. (Photograph by kind permission of Mr B. Wessier, Silver Medallist in the Disabled Olympic Games, New York, 1984.)

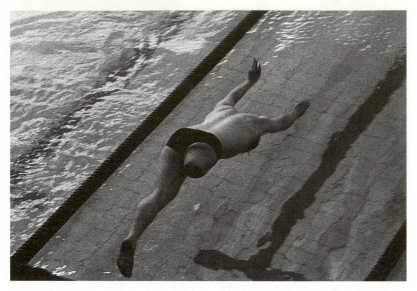

Fig. 15.2   An above-knee amputee diving into a swimming pool. (Photograph by kind permission of Mr D. Breakwell.)

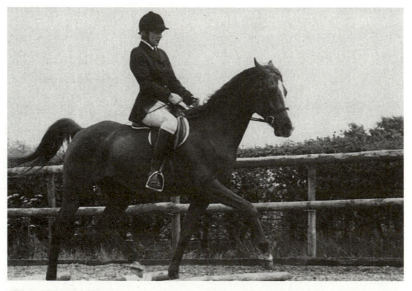

Fig. 15.3   A below-knee amputee horse riding, with an adapted boot. (Photograph by kind permission of Mrs J. Upton.)

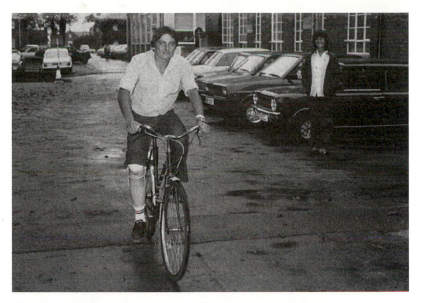

Fig. 15.4   A below-knee amputee, wearing a temporary prosthesis, learning to bicycle in the DSC car park.

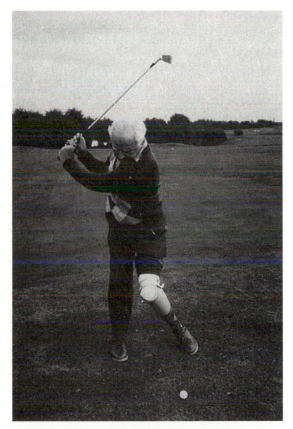

Fig. 15.5   A below-knee amputee playing golf.
(Photograph by kind permission of Mr P. Everett.)

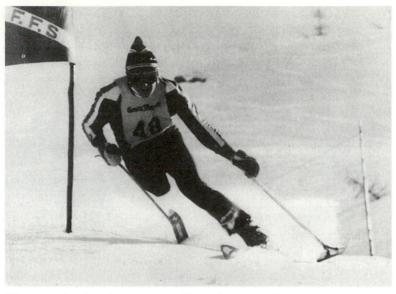

Fig. 15.6 An above-knee amputee skiing using poles with outriggers. (Photograph by kind permission of Mr M. Hammond.)

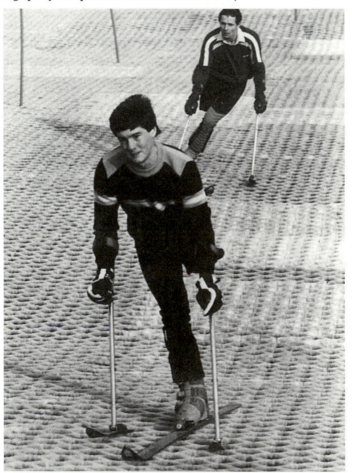

Fig. 15.7 A young above-knee amputee learning to ski on a dry ski slope with an instructor, Mr M. Hammond, who is also an amputee. (Photograph by kind permission of the Harlow Gazette.)

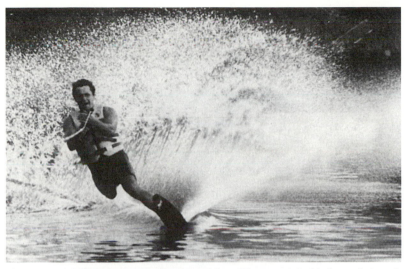

Fig. 15.8   An above-knee amputee water skiing. (Photograph by kind permission of Mr M. Hammond.)

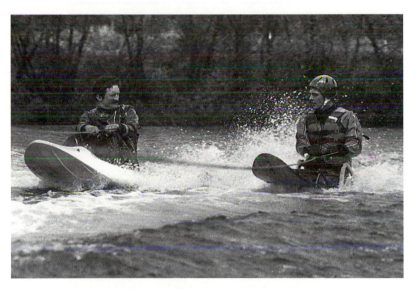

Fig. 15.9   A bilateral amputee (on the right) water skiing with an instructor. (Photograph by kind permission of Mr Berkeley and Mr I. D. Hassall.)

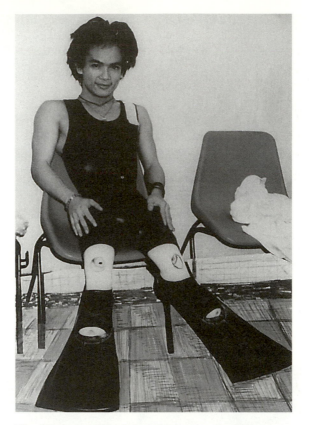

Fig. 15.10   A bilateral above-knee amputee with custom-made 'fin legs'. (Photograph by kind permission of Mr Long Tran and Therapy Weekly.)

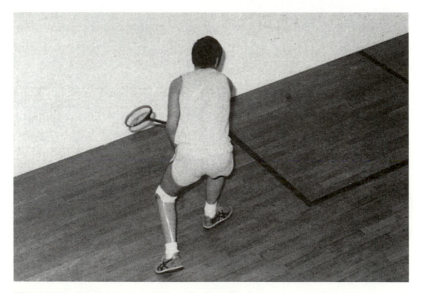

Fig. 15.11   A below-knee amputee playing squash.

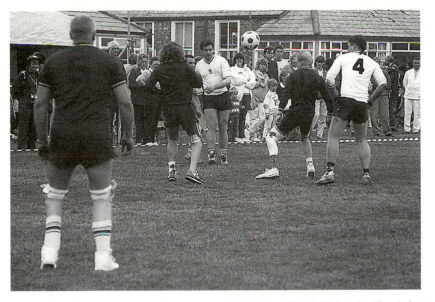

Fig. 15.12   A demonstration football match at the Queen Mary's University Hospital annual garden party. (Photograph by kind permission of Ms J. Jackson.)

The amputee may have a spare prosthesis which the prosthetist may like to experiment with before fabricating an individual special prosthesis, which is a costly undertaking. This prosthesis can then be tried to see if it helps with a specific sporting activity.

REFERENCES

Burgess E M, Hittenberger D A, Forsgren S M, Lindh D V 1983 The Seattle Prosthetic Foot — A design for active sports: preliminary studies. Orthotics and Prosthetics 37(1): 25–31

Gailey R 1992 Recreational pursuits for elders with amputation. Topics in Geriatric Rehabilitation 8(1): 39–58.

Gailey R, Stinson D 1991 Analysis of above-knee running gait. Proceedings, World Confederation of Physical Therapy 11th International Congress.

Hittenberger D A 1982 Extra-ambulatory activities and the amputee. Clinical Prosthetics and Orthotics 6(4): 1 – 4

Kegel B 1986 Journal of Rehabilitation Research and Development: Clinical Supplement No 1. Veterans Administration USA

Kegel B, Carpenter M L, Burgess E M 1978 Functional capabilities of lower extremity amputees. Archives of Physical Medicine and Rehabilitation 59: 109–119

Levesque C, Gautier-Gagnon C 1987 An above-knee prosthesis for rock climbing. Orthotics and Prosthetics 40(1): 41–45

Rubin G, Fleiss D 1983 Devices to enable persons with amputation to participate in sports. Archives of Physical Medicine and Rehabilitation 64: 37–40

Sports Activities 1978 Physiotherapy 64 (10): 290–301, (11): 324–329

16. Bilateral amputees

The rehabilitation potential of the bilateral amputee depends on the underlying pathology, the extent of any other disease process present, and the patient's motivation. The ablation of both lower limbs is a devastating experience and great tact and sympathy of approach is needed from the whole team, both when treating the patient and when talking to the relatives and carers.

Acceptance of the situation by the patient can take time, which in turn may slow down rehabilitation. This period of adjustment is vital. While recovery and adjustment are taking place, the team must be planning ahead for the patient's future management.

It is known that 30% of single amputees suffering from peripheral vascular disease (PVD) will become bilateral amputees within 3 years. Those single amputees who have walked well up until a few weeks before the second amputation have a good chance of successful prosthetic rehabilitation. However, those single amputees who are chairfast because of pain in the remaining leg, will be less generally fit and will always take much longer to rehabilitate. There is also a small group of patients with PVD who have both legs amputated simultaneously. Apart from experiencing the obvious psychological shock, the patient is also systemically ill and recovery may take many weeks. Rehabilitation for this group of amputees will take longer.

Patients who become bilateral amputee because of gross trauma are few in number. Although these patients encounter the same problems as the vascular group, the systemic problems of progressive disease are not present. Once recovery and rehabilitation are complete, the patient's po-

tential is much greater since there is no limitation from cardiorespiratory dysfunction.

Pre-operative treatment

Unilateral amputees suffering from PVD and admitted to hospital for further vascular or diabetic investigation should be monitored by the ward physiotherapist. Their physical condition may well have deteriorated markedly since they were last seen by a physiotherapist, and joint contractures, muscle weakness and deterioration in the condition of the remaining foot may present a problem. In order to maintain patients as single amputees for as long as possible, it may be necessary to start an exercise programme for those confined to bed, or to assess patients for general mobility and possibly make specialist footwear (e.g. a Plastazote shoe), provide walking aids or alter the prosthetic fit.

If it becomes apparent that a second amputation is likely, then a full assessment is required. The most important factor here is the home situation. This has to be considered in a different manner from the assessment for the single amputee. Is the home suitable or adaptable for a wheelchair and is help at hand in the house? The most effective way of initially assessing this is to carry out a home visit taking just the wheelchair: the patient does not need to attend at this stage. The social worker may need to be contacted immediately with regard to finding future placement or rehousing and involving relatives if difficulties are apparent.

Relevant goal setting in a realistic time frame is the key to managing the bilateral amputee. Many are unlikely to be able to walk with any degree of functional independence and false hopes must be avoided. Rehabilitation takes a long time, often many months, and involves a large team of professionals, carers and relatives. It may be more realistic to transfer the patient after surgery to a specialist centre, which is able to provide this time and resource.

All bilateral amputees will require a wheelchair, (see Ch. 5), irrespective of their age, condition and level of amputation. This wheelchair must have the rear wheels set back 7.5 cm to compensate for the alteration is weight distribution of the patient in the chair, owing to the loss of both lower limbs. If the amputee already possesses a wheelchair which does not conform to these requirements, it must be changed.

Physiotherapy techniques employed at this stage involve the teaching of independent transfers, without the patient using the remaining leg (see Figs 3.9 and 3.10), and the strengthening of upper limbs and trunk within the limits of the patient's medical condition and pain tolerance.

Postoperative treatment

In the first few postoperative days it is difficult for the bilateral amputee to move about in bed. The standard high/low bed should have been prepared pre-operatively with cot sides, monkey pole and pressure area relief aids (see Ch. 2). The essential activities which need to be taught by the physiotherapist from the *first postoperative day* are:

1. Sitting up in bed
2. Balance
3. Bed mobility
4. Transfers.

Sitting up in bed

This must be achieved by the patient pushing down on the bed with the arms one at a time and rotating the trunk a quarter turn to one side then a quarter turn to the other (see Fig. 3.3).

The monkey pole is only useful for bilateral amputees for lifting up onto bedpans and for pressure area care.

Balance

It is very common for bilateral amputees (particularly those with higher level amputations) to overbalance backwards. Rhythmic stabilisations in unsupported sitting are the most useful exercises. Manual resistance should initially be applied to the trunk; when balance is achieved in this manner, the resistance is then applied distally to the patient's outstretched arms.

Bed mobility

This is best achieved by the patient hip hitching in upright sitting, and moving each buttock alternately. Forwards, backwards and sideways 'walking' on the buttocks is practised. Some patients with short arms require push-up blocks in order to achieve this mobility (see Fig. 4.2).

Transfers

Backwards transfer off the bed into a suitable wheelchair (with stump boards where necessary) is taught (see Fig. 3.9).

Success in these early activities and future potential for independent mobility will be based on four physical considerations:

— *Muscle strength*: good upper limb and trunk strength, as well as balance, will determine ease of mobility.
— *Trunk mobility*: a full range of movement in the joints and general flexibility is needed.
— *Body proportions*: those patients with a long trunk and short arms, and those with large abdomens, will find mobility difficult.
— *Medical condition*: cardiovascular status, level of cerebral function and rate of deterioration in progressive conditions will also affect mobility.

Exercise programme

The patient then progresses to an exercise programme in the physiotherapy department as outlined in Chapter 4, as it is much easier to assess and treat the patient on a firm wide plinth. At this stage the patient must be dressed. Dressing practice with the occupational therapist is a crucial activity, particularly for the lower half of the body and clothing adaptations may be necessary. The ability to dress will be a strong indicator of the patient's ability to don the prosthesis.

Rolling is an excellent activity for both function and exercise. Once strength and confidence have been gained, further exercise can be done by the patient on a mat on the floor (Fig. 16.1). Here, for the fitter, more active patient, free active exercise can be carried out quickly and energetically, without the fear of falling. This is usually more popular with men than women. Games can be fun and competitive: adapted badminton, hockey, netball, etc. are all of value. Hydrotherapy is also a useful therapeutic activity.

Single below-knee amputees who were competent prosthetic users may be able to use the existing prosthesis after becoming bilateral amputees, for transfers and limited mobility. Some patients can regard this as their 'normal' leg, managing standing pivot transfers (see Ch. 3) and hopping a few steps in the parallel bars. However, a single through-knee or above-knee amputee who was competent on a prosthesis before becoming a bilateral amputee will not be able to use the existing prosthesis for mobility. These patients may use this prosthesis for comfort, cosmesis and psychological reassurance when sitting in the wheelchair.

Great caution must be observed in the use of the Ppam aid with bilateral amputees. If the first amputation was at the below-knee level and the patient was a good prosthetic user, a Ppam aid on the second stump can be used along with the existing prosthesis. Standing and walking should only be attempted for short periods of time (up to half an hour per day) in the parallel bars under the close supervision of the physiotherapist. If walking is unsuccessful, it may be that the patient is too tall and the Ppam aid is unstable on the stump, making the leverage difficult. The Ppam aid is more useful as an additional assessment tool for the bilateral amputee, rather than for oedema control, pre-prosthetic preparation of the stump and walking. Two Ppam aids should never be used, because of lack of stability, pistoning and possible damage to the wounds. Lack of success using the Ppam aid, however, does not necessarily mean that the patient is unsuitable for prostheses. Femuretts, however, provide more support and may be more suitable for the bilateral amputee.

The occupational therapist will also be seeing the patient regularly for activities of daily living practice, and the social worker will be seeing the patient and carers for both counselling and service arrangements. A composite picture of the patient's potential will gradually emerge, and a case conference is the best way to determine the bilateral amputee's suitability for limb fitting. The general considerations outlined in Chapter 6 should be referred to; however, it must be remembered that this decision can be changed at any time if the patient's condition or circumstances alter.

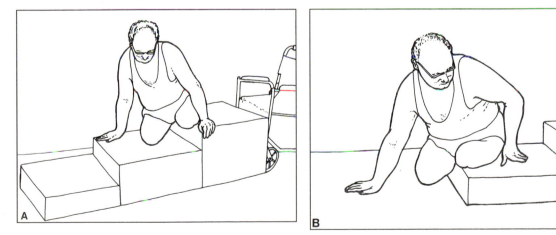

Fig. 16.1   A bilateral above-knee amputee transferring from wheelchair to floor using graded box heights.

The prosthetic rehabilitation procedure

After full assessment by the hospital rehabilitation team (see Ch. 6), bilateral amputees will be referred on to the local DSC; this will be a familiar procedure for some, as they will have already attended as single amputees. For others, however, this first visit may be quite bemusing.

A detailed medical, rehabilitation and social assessment, including a home visit report, should accompany the patient in order for the team at the DSC to understand the individual patient's situation.

Prostheses supplied to bilateral amputees are generally reduced in height to lower the patient's centre of gravity so that ability to balance is retained. Careful explanation of this must be given.

Considerable time is needed to rehabilitate patients using two prostheses, and regular sessions in a physiotherapy department are required. It is preferable that bilateral amputees attend a unit with a prosthetist in attendance because often many small adjustments to the sockets need to be made.

Prosthetic rehabilitation can extend in time up to 2 months or more. If, however, after a month of regular attendances, there is little sign of improvement, the physiotherapist, doctor and patient must seriously consider whether it is worth the patient continuing trying to walk. Many bilateral amputees, especially those with the higher levels of amputation, are unrealistic about their future capabilities using prostheses. It may be important that these patients have the opportunity to try, but, if they are unsuccessful, the team and the amputee must decide when they should stop. It may then be appropriate to supply cosmetic prostheses for wheelchair use (see Fig. 6.1A & B) and other rehabilitation goals are explored. Independance and activity do not solely depend on the use of prostheses.

THE BILATERAL ABOVE-KNEE AMPUTEE

These patients usually commence walking using short rocker pylons (SRP) (see Fig. 16.2). The pylons are usually 46 cm from the ischial seating to the floor; there are no articulations at the knee joints and the base consists of a backward facing rocker. The rocker is designed so that the

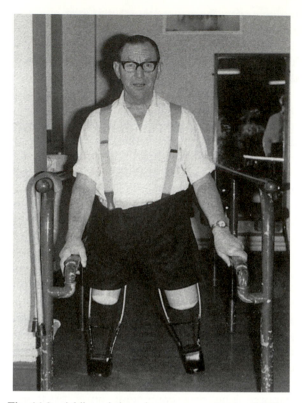

Fig. 16.2 A bilateral above-knee amputee wearing the fiirst stage short rocker pylons. Note the height of parallel bar required.

patient's centre of gravity always falls inside the area of support of the base when the patient is walking. It also helps to prevent the patient from falling backwards and assists in forward propulsion. The sockets are ischial weightbearing and usually made of metal, and the suspension consists of two rigid pelvic bands (RPBs) with posterior and anterior fastenings. Shoulder straps may or may not be necessary.

The supply of prostheses will depend upon the patient's ability and mobility (see Ch. 11). Not all bilateral above-knee amputees reach this stage of prostheses; some remain at the SRP stage. Generally, it takes some months from the date of the second amputation to reach the stage of functional independence with prostheses.

Application of SRPs and prostheses

It takes time to learn how to put on and take off prostheses, and the bilateral amputee must be able to carry this out independently at home. If this is too difficult and tiring, the amputee will become disenchanted with the whole process of using prostheses and will probably give up.

The following instructions should be given to the patient (see Fig. 16.3):

1. Transfer forwards onto a large solid bed the same height as the wheelchair seat, e.g. a

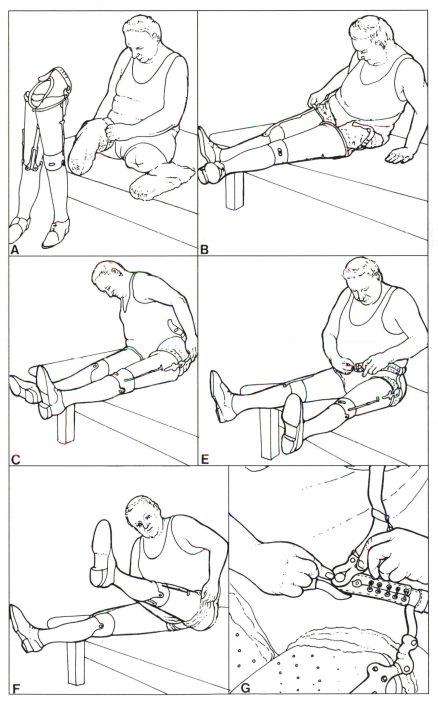

Fig. 16.3 Application of prostheses by a bilateral above-knee amputee.

Bobath plinth. Do not use a narrow high bed, as it is both dangerous and frightening. (Later on the patient must also repeat this activity on a fairly soft narrow bed, similar to that at home, before discharge from rehabilitation.)

2. Undress so that only a long vest is worn. (Men prefer to keep their underpants on. Women will either have to put their pants on over the prostheses, or not wear underwear, in order that they can use the toilet.)

3. Pull on stump socks (see Fig. 16.3A)

4. Position the prostheses on the bed within arms reach. The shoulder straps should be attached posteriorly and the RPBs should be fastened posteriorly.

5. Gradually ease the stumps into the socket, at the same time pulling the RPBs back up over the buttocks onto the hips. This may be carried out by the patient rolling from buttock to buttock pulling alternately on the RPBs (Fig. 16.3B and C). Or the patient may prefer to push up on the hands and lift the trunk up over the fastened RPBs and then pull belts up over the buttocks to the hip level (Fig. 16.3D).

6. Once the RPBs are in the correct position, the anterior fastening should be secured (Fig. 16.3E).

7. The stump socks should be pulled up and turned down over the rim of the sockets (Fig. 16.3F). It may be necessary to secure the stump sock around the upright of the hip joint using a safety pin.

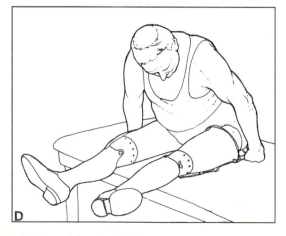

Fig. 16.3 (cont'd)   Application of prosthesis by a bilateral above-knee amputee.

8. The shoulder straps should be fastened at the front (see Fig. 16.3G). These should be crossed at the back and adjusted when standing so that the correct tension is achieved (see Ch. 11).

9. Transfer backwards into the wheelchair, as it is easier to stand up from a chair with arms than from the bed.

After the first few attempts at applying the prostheses, the patient is then taught to dress the prostheses with trousers first (if worn). Once the prostheses are on the patient, it is exceptionally difficult to thread them into trouser legs.

Some bilateral amputees are too rotund and find it impossible to apply the prostheses with the RPBs fastened posteriorly. In these cases, it is necessary to put on each prosthesis separately and then fasten the RPBs at the back afterwards. This is only possible if there is a Velcro and D-ring, or a large buckle fastening, and even then it may be impossible to fasten this independently. For correct alignment of the prostheses, the posterior fastening must be secured in exactly the same position each time.

Sometimes amputees at the short rocker pylon stage are encouraged to apply the pylons by sitting in a chair or on a bed and sliding down into the standing sockets. This usually means that another person has to hold the prostheses steady for this procedure. This is not a very safe method and the patient does not learn how to apply the prostheses independently. Furthermore, this method is impossible in the later stages with longer prostheses.

For comfort, some men may need to wear a scrotal support as the medial brims of the sockets may be close together.

Check of the prostheses

This is first carried out with the bilateral amputee seated. The RPBs must be comfortable, and the anterior brim of the socket must not impinge upon the soft tissues of the abdomen. The patient then stands supported by a standing frame or parallel bars. The fit of the sockets, the suspension, the alignment and the correct length is checked (see Ch. 11). Rotation of the rocker bases or feet is determined by adjusting the RPBs. If the posterior fastening is too tight, the bases will be excessively externally rotated. This can be adjusted by releasing the posterior fastening and tightening the anterior fastenings. If, however, the bases are too internally rotated, the posterior fastening should be tightened and the anterior fastening released.

It is often worth waiting for several sessions before attempting many adjustments, or telephoning the prosthetist for assistance, as it takes several days for the new bilateral amputee to become used to wearing two hard sockets. Several treatment sessions are often required for the patient to learn to stand up straight, and this may have a direct bearing on the physiotherapist's opinion concerning the correct length of the prostheses. Incorrect length is apparent when the patient is unable to initiate swing phase and hitch the prosthesis clear of the floor.

Walking

Walking must always commence in the parallel bars at whatever stage of prosthetic fitting. Special low bars are required for those with short rocker pylons (see Fig. 16.2). At first the physiotherapist should stand behind patients and gently rock them backwards and forwards, so that they become used to the rocking motion in standing. The patient is then encouraged to stand as straight as possible during this exercise. Once this is achieved the patient is encouraged to rock from side to side, gradually learning to hitch the non-weightbearing socket up each time. Patients can then progress to stepping forwards. After that, walking starts: the pattern is wide based, giving the amputee greater stability. A most common habit, observed with all bilateral amputees, is forward flexion at the hips. This should be corrected as much as possible by teaching the patient to extend the hip and lower trunk when weightbearing. However much both the patient and the physiotherapist try to correct this, it often remains, and the amputee tends to walk using a flexed action, relying heavily on walking aids for support. This is a balance and mobility problem, and in many cases it is not related to hip flexion contractures.

During the stages of prosthetic rehabilitation,

the bilateral above-knee amputee will initially walk with a stiff knee gait pattern on both prostheses. This involves alternate hip hitching and is often slow and laborious with a wide base. A degree of circumduction is inevitable.

The gait pattern at the later stage will depend very much upon the prescription of the knee mechanisms supplied. Generally, the amputee learns to walk with one knee stiff and one free. Occasionally, if the bilateral above-knee amputee is extremely fit, young and mobile, it is possible to walk with a more natural gait pattern.

Progression to aids

As soon as the patient is mobile and balanced within the parallel bars, progression is made to suitable walking aids; either walking sticks or tetrapods should be used. Those patients who have a good sense of balance and are reasonably mobile can progress to two sticks. Those who are flexed and find walking rather laborious, require two tetrapods. Occasionally patients manage with one stick and one tetrarapod; if at all possible this is preferable, as it reduces the space required to manoeuvre.

It is extremely inadvisable for any bilateral amputee to use a walking frame. The action of lifting the frame up and moving it forwards alters the centre of gravity in bilateral amputees and disturbs their sense of balance; consequently, they tend to fall backwards. The width of the frame restricts the walking base, and the rocking action of the amputee often tips the frame sideways, and although the frames are supportive they can be dangerous if the amputee falls.

Getting up from a chair

The choice of chair is important. It must have strong arms which extend to the edge of the seat and be of sufficient height to enable the patient to push into standing. Care must be taken to ensure that the chair will not slide backwards as the patient pushes on it to stand up. The bilateral amputee's own wheelchair is often the most suitable as it has the advantages of brakes and stability. It must also be wide enough to enable the amputee to stand up without catching the suspension or sockets on the arms of the chair. In some cases, if the patient is wide, it may be necessary to order an extra-wide chair, or outset the front fixing slot of the arm rests to accommodate this problem. The height of the chair may have to change if the length of the prostheses alters.

With short rocker pylons

The following instructions should be given to the patient:

1. Ease bottom forward until the posterior edges of the rocker bases are touching the floor.
2. Push up on the arms of the chair, extending the elbows; at the same time pull or walk the bases backwards, until they are in total contact with the floor. (At this stage the patient's bottom should be off the seat of the chair.)
3. Continue pushing on the arms of the chair, rocking onto the bases of the SRPs, until an upright position is achieved. NB: At the moment of push up from the chair the patient must transfer his weight from the arms of the chair onto walking aids. This action may be carried out straight from the chair, or at an angle. The patient may well feel very unsafe at this moment.

If the bilateral amputee is using walking sticks, these must be held in each hand at the beginning of this pushing up movement. Those amputees using tetrarapods find it easier to stand up, as the aids are free-standing and can be grasped once the amputee is in the upright position.

This method may also be used for short patients with short prostheses.

With prostheses (see Fig. 16.4)

1. Straighten one knee.
2. Twist the trunk on the seat of the chair towards the flexed knee (Fig. 16.4A).
3. Ease the body forward so that the foot of the prosthesis with the flexed knee is in total contact with the floor.
4. Push up on hands on the arms of the chair, extending the elbows; the body is still slightly towards one side, and the bottom should be off the chair seat (Fig. 16.4B).
5. At this stage extend the stump with the flexed

knee. The hand on the side of the stiff knee must push off from the arm of the chair and come forwards using the stick for support (Fig. 16.4C).
6. As soon as balance is achieved, remove the second hand from the chair and take weight through the second stick. Stand fully upright (Fig. 16.4D).

This is a more difficult method, but it has to be utilised if the prostheses are too long for the amputee to push up into a standing position while facing forwards as with SRPs.

Success with either of these procedures depends on the length of the prostheses and how this relates to the length of the patient's arms and trunk. If the patient cannot carry out either method, the physiotherapist must decide if the prostheses are too long. Often the height and length of chair arms must be altered or it will be necessary to contact the prosthetist so that the prostheses can be shortened.

Unless standing up from a chair can be achieved independently with ease and safety a bilateral amputee is unlikely to walk.

Sitting down in a chair

The methods described above apply here but in reverse order. The most important aspect is that the amputee aligns his body with the chair correctly. Many amputees try to sit down at an angle, grabbing one arm rest; this invariably tips the chair, making the whole procedure unsafe. Many position themselves so closely to the seat of the chair that they become wedged, with the bases or feet jammed on the floor and the trunk jammed against the seat. This is very uncomfortable, and the patient has to be taught how to gauge the distance correctly.

Toilet

Bilateral above-knee amputees need to organise their bladder and bowel habits; using the toilet whilst wearing the prostheses may be difficult, unhygienic and uncomfortable.

Men like to stand to urinate and many are able to use their prostheses for this, but for a bowel motion it is preferable not to wear prostheses.

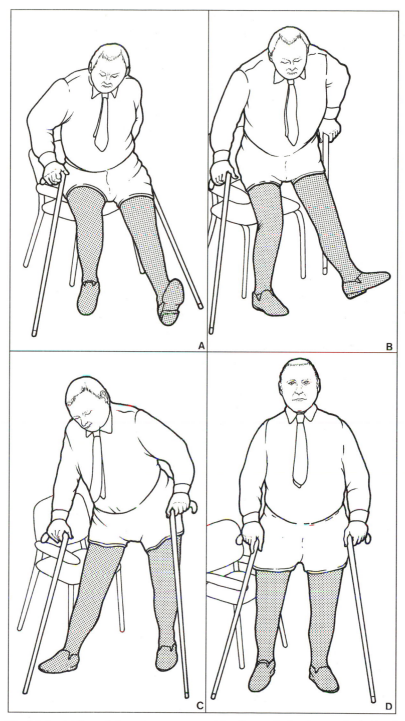

Fig. 16.4 A bilateral above-knee amputee rising from a chair using one locked and one free knee mechanism.

Women generally prefer not to use the prostheses for either bladder or bowel motion, and for some women this inconvenience may determine whether they continue to use prostheses at all.

Independence in the application of the prostheses, standing up from a chair, walking and using the toilet are the basic goals that the bilateral above-knee amputee must achieve if prosthetic use is to be possible. In many cases this is all that the physiotherapist and patient can hope to achieve, even with great effort, determination and hard work on all sides.

The following activities will only be achieved by the younger, fitter, more agile and determined patient.

Stairs

Although two methods are illustrated here (Figs 16.5 and 16.6), variations may need to be worked out for different individuals, depending on their ability and the type of stairs they have at home.

Initially, a method is taught using two bannisters until strength and safety have been achieved. Progress to one stick and one bannister may be possible, but walking upstairs using two sticks is usually impossible for the bilateral above-knee amputee. The safety of any bannisters to be used, either in a physiotherapy department or at home, must be checked, as the force and leverage exerted on them is considerable.

Slopes

These are much more difficult than stairs. A very wide-based gait is used (Fig. 16.7). Initially, a very gentle incline with a handrail is used, with progression to steeper inclines and two walking aids if possible.

Kerb or step

This is the most difficult obstacle for the bilateral above-knee amputee. The correct starting position is vital; the patient should stand as close as possible to the step (see Figs 16.8 and 16.9). Coordination, weight transference, balance and arm strength are all necessary. the ability to climb up a step also depends on the height of the step and the length of the prostheses.

Progression to a kerb outside in the street is not easy for the bilateral amputee, as the camber of the gutter, any drain covers, yellow lines (as these are raised and slippery), as well as the worry of passing traffic and pushing pedestrians, make the kerb more difficult to negotiate.

Getting up from the floor

The method illustrated (Fig. 16.10) can only be used by the exceptionally fit bilateral above-knee

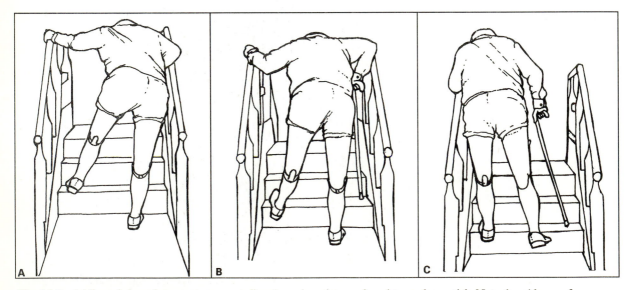

Fig. 16.5   A bilateral above-knee amputee ascending the stairs using one bannister and one stick. Note the wide arc of movement of the pelvis and trunk.

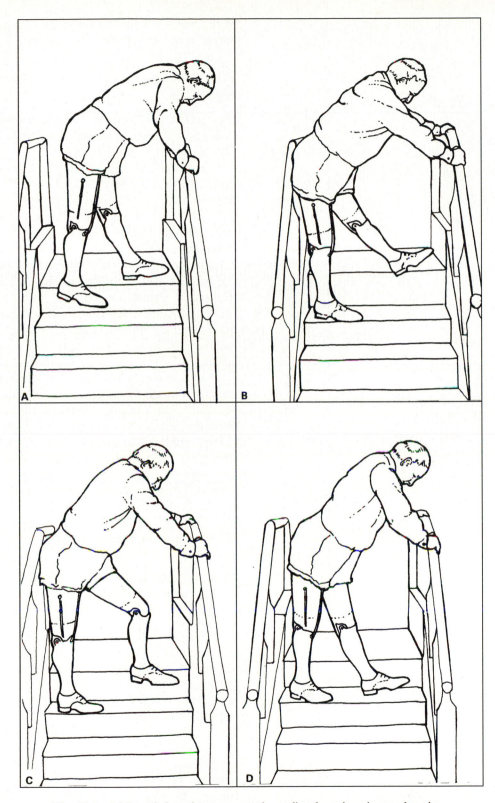

Fig. 16.6   A bilateral above-knee amputee descending the stairs using one bannister.

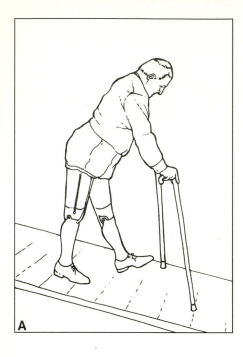

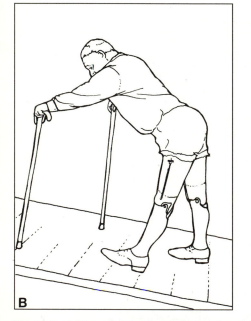

Fig. 16.7   A bilateral above-knee amputee descending (A) and ascending (B) a slope. Note the amount of forward flexion required in (B).

amputee, and not by the PVD patient. Those amputees unable to succeed with this method must either enlist the help of two strong people or remove the prostheses and try to get up using arm strength and items of furniture.

THE BILATERAL THROUGH-KNEE AMPUTEE

Hip flexion contractures are disastrous for these patients and may preclude prosthetic use (see Ch. 11).

The method of application of the prostheses is similar to that for the bilateral above-knee level, but obviously the sockets and suspension may be different (see Ch. 12). Rehabilitation follows the same pattern as that described for the bilateral above-knee level.

It is possible for a bilateral through-knee amputee to walk directly on the weightbearing stumps, if these are covered with protective Plastazote boots (see Fig. 6.2). These can be made by the physiotherapist or occupational therapist. It is important that the wounds have healed well and that the stumps can tolerate pressure before the amputee commences walking directly on the stumps, using tetrapods. Occasionally, for those patients who are unable to use prostheses, these stump boots (sometimes called elephant boots) can be made by the prosthetist out of materials such as blocked leather. This enables the patient to walk in the home, permitting access to the toilet and bathroom and spaces too small for the wheelchair to negotiate. The patient can also walk outside with these boots in order to transfer into a car.

THE BELOW-KNEE AND THROUGH-KNEE OR ABOVE-KNEE COMBINATION

The presence of one natural knee joint can speed up and facilitate rehabilitation, enabling the bilateral amputee to achieve greater levels of activity and mobility. However, if there is a problem with the natural knee joint, or if the stump is unhealed, or breaks down as a result of forces exerted on it, it will be a hindrance.

Pre-prosthetically, balance and movement in the bed can be as difficult for these patients as for other bilateral amputees. The below-knee stump tends to be pushed hard into the mattress and soreness or wound breakdown can result.

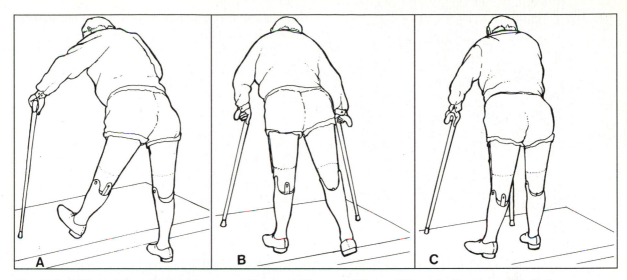

Fig. 16.8 A bilateral above-knee amputee ascending a step using two stiff knees. This method is only possible for low steps.

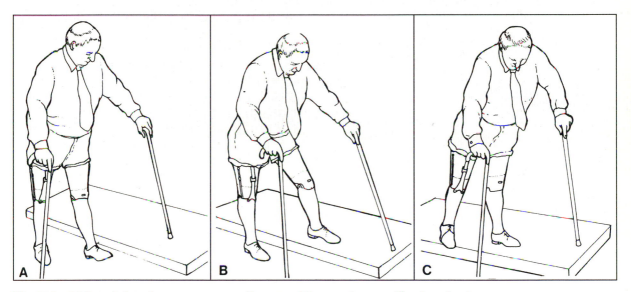

Fig. 16.9 A bilateral above-knee amputee ascending a step sideways using one stiff and one free knee.

The speed of rehabilitation depends on whether the below-knee amputation was performed first or second. If it was performed first, and prosthetic rehabilitation had been achieved with this level of amputation, the situation is easier. If it was performed second, then the below-knee stump is more liable to serious damage, as it will tend to be used more than the contralateral side, both pre-prosthetically and subsequently with the prosthesis.

The patient learns to apply the prostheses, using a wide plinth the same height as the wheel-chair seat, but each prosthesis is applied separately.

For prosthetic rehabilitation, the below-knee side may be regarded as a normal leg; this gives the patient a greater chance of being able to manage steps, stairs, slopes and rough ground. These activities will cause considerable stress to the tissues of the below-knee stump, particularly during the early stages. The physiotherapist must

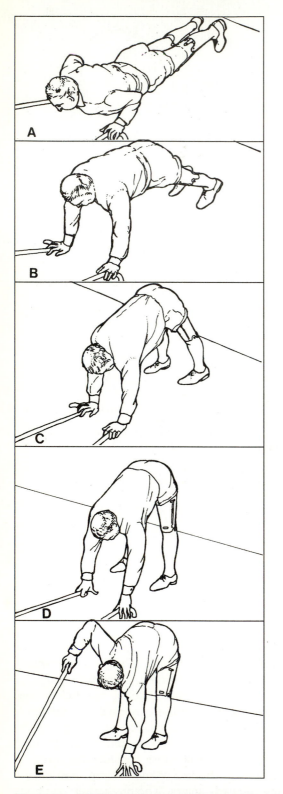

Fig. 16.10 A bilateral above-knee amputee getting up from the floor. Note the amount of trunk and hip mobility required.

frequently check the skin for redness, soreness or abrasions (see Ch. 13).

Even with one natural knee joint present, the patient's height may be reduced to improve balance.

THE BILATERAL BELOW-KNEE AMPUTEE

Nearly all bilateral below-knee amputees are supplied with prostheses, and they can expect to be able to walk and become independent, within their capabilities, irrespective of their age and condition. Despite this, a wheelchair is always necessary for all bilateral below-knee amputees for toileting and washing, morning and evening, and for travelling distances. Initially, the skin of the stumps will not tolerate long walking distances and a slow and gradual build up of tissue tolerance to weightbearing must be allowed. Again, as with all bilateral amputees, the overall height of the patient will be reduced.

Occasionally, an above-knee/below-knee temporary prosthesis may be supplied initially. Although rehabilitation with one free knee and one locked knee produces a slow, uneven gait pattern, it is worth the wait for wound healing and the prospect of two PTBs being fitted in the future.

During gait re-education with the physiotherapist, frequent checks must be made on the skin (see Ch. 13). Although the patient gains independence quickly and may be capable of walking with sticks at an early stage, attention to skin problems must be uppermost in the physiotherapist's mind. Initially, treatment sessions may be very short, with frequent rests. Frank breakdown of the skin or opening of the wound is a disaster and can happen within a very short time, possibly 1 hour, if care is not taken.

Application of the prostheses is not difficult: the method is described in Chapter 13. It is advisable that the patient learns to apply the prostheses on a bed, as well as in the chair. Occasionally, patients wearing two PTBs may need pick-up straps from the supracondylar cuffs to a waist belt to improve the suspension (see Fig. 13.4). If the patient was an established user of a conventional thigh corset prosthesis before the second amputation, it is possible that this prescription may be kept but a PTB supplied for the newer stump.

The walking aids most commonly used for this level of amputation are a pair of walking sticks, and many patients progress to using one stick once the stumps have matured. Obstacles such as stairs, slopes, steps and rough ground can be negotiated by most, including the elderly. It is advisable for the patient to use a chair with arm rests, which will assist push-up to standing. Getting up after a fall, or from the floor, can be managed by kneeling before standing.

THE BILATERAL HIP DISARTICULATION

This extremely severe and mutilating level of amputation is rarely seen. The two most important rehabilitative goals for the patient to achieve are sitting balance and transfers. A sitting 'shell' or a special seating material, e.g. a Matrix system, may be useful for balance and can be made at the local wheelchair clinic. Cosmetic prostheses can be attached to this seat so that normal body image is maintained.

If the patient wishes to walk and the team assessment is such that this is possible, prostheses are supplied which provide a swing through gait with locked knees (similar to a paraplegic gait). The patient must have very strong arms and trunk muscles, good balance, a mobile lumbar spine and great determination.

It is difficult for the patient to apply the prostheses at this level and almost impossible to stand up from a chair independently.

PROSTHESES INFORMATION

Detailed information regarding prostheses available in the UK can be obtained from the manufacturers. The addresses are listed in the Appendix.

REFERENCES

DuBow L L, Witt P L, Kadaba M P, Reynes R, Cochran G V B 1983 Oxygen consumption of elderly persons with bilateral knee amputations: ambulation vs wheelchair propulsion. Archives of Physical Medicine and Rehabilitation 64: 255–259

Kerstein M D, Zimmer H, Dugdale F E, Lerner 1975 Associated diagnoses which complicate rehabilitation of the patient with bilateral lower extremity amputations. Surgery, Gynaecology and Obstetrics 140: 875–876

McCollough N C 1972 The bilateral lower extremity amputee. Orthopedic Clinics of North America 3(2): 373–382

McCollough N C, Jennings J J, Sarmiento A 1972 Bilateral below-the-knee amputation in patients over fifty years of age. Journal of Bone and Joint Surgery 54A(6): 1217–1223

Moverly L 1990 Discovering water's redeeming features. Therapy Weekly 17(7): 4

Muthu S 1983 Limb fitting and survival in the dysvascular double above-knee amputee. Journal of the Royal College of Surgeons of Edinburgh 28(3): 157–159

Svetz W R 1983 A novel concept in fitting bilateral above-knee amputees: a case history. Orthotics and Prosthetics 37(3): 63–66

Van de Ven C M C 1973 A pilot survey of elderly bilateral lower-limb amputees. Physiotherapy 59(10): 316–320

Van de Ven C M C 1981 An investigation into the management of bilateral leg amputees. British Medical Journal 283:707

Volpicelli L J, Chambers R B, Wagner F W 1983 Ambulation levels of bilateral lower-extremity amputees. Journal of Bone and Joint Surgery 65A(5): 599–604

Wolf E et al 1989 Prosthetic rehabilitation of elderly bilateral amputees. International Journal of Rehabilitation Research 12(3): 271–278

17. Upper limb amputation and congenital limb deficiency

Alicia Mendez OBE, FCOT, revised by Fiona Carnegie DipCOT

The ratio of upper to lower limb amputation is very low (approximately 1 : 24). The number of primary upper limb amputees and limb-deficient children registered annually in the UK is approximately 330, which accounts for about 6% of all primary amputees. It is not surprising, therefore, that few cases are seen in any one hospital. However, it is important that any hospital department is able to carry out the initial treatment required before the patient moves on to the prosthetic stage, attending a Disablement Services Centre (DSC) and the Occupational Therapy Department for full prosthetic rehabilitation.

There are two distinct groups of clients requiring upper limb prostheses: those with an acquired amputation, and those with congenital limb deficiency. There are major differences in the management of these two groups because of the nature of the disabilities and age disparities (see Table 1.3).

Acquired amputation

Trauma

This is usually the result of a road traffic accident, industrial injury, a severe domestic accident, explosion or gunshot wounds. Amputation for trauma is normally seen in the adolescent and adult working population where exposure to trauma is more likely to occur. The incidence is greater in men than women because of the differing nature of their work. The number of traumatic arm amputations has reduced over the past 10–15 years. The Health and Safety at Work Act 1974 has resulted in workplaces becoming safer; sociological changes mean that fewer people are working in industrial environments and more

are working in less hazardous office-based jobs. For those who do have traumatic hand injuries, microsurgery techniques have improved, resulting in the hand sometimes being saved.

Traumatic amputation of the upper limb may also occur in children and the elderly, but this is uncommon.

Disease

Malignant tumours, leprosy and thrombosis/embolism come into this category. General vascular insufficiency, such as peripheral vascular disease, is very rarely a cause for upper limb amputation, but occasionally patients with severe Buerger's or Raynaud's disease may require an amputation.

Amputation because of disease can take place at any age, but it is frequently seen in the young adult. Improved treatment in the field of oncology has helped prolong the lifespan of such patients, but the long-term prognosis is still not good and the earliest possible intervention for prosthetic fitting and rehabilitation is therefore very important. The patient with thrombosis or embolism has a good prognosis following amputation.

Congenital limb deficiency

These are rare within the whole amputee population but form 40% of all primary upper limb referrals per year. Specialised treatment techniques are required, with constant review, particularly throughout growth and development in childhood and adolescence.

The reasons for congenital limb deformity remain obscure. Apart from the thalidomide tragedy in the early 1960s, the number of children born each year with these deformities remains relatively constant at 1 : 10 000 live births. Genetic research continues, and knowledge of the time at which cells are formed for limbs in utero indicates that, whatever the reason, the malformation happens early in the pregnancy.

The treatment procedures for these two distinct groups of patients will be divided into two sections for clarity: acquired amputation, and congenital deficiencies.

ACQUIRED AMPUTATION

Usually there is no opportunity for pre-amputation consultations as the amputation occurs at the time of the accident or immediately afterwards.

It is helpful for the patient's future management when such a consultation can be carried out, e.g. in the case of an amputation as a result of disease, or when surgical intervention has been unable to create a functional hand. In the latter case there may be an element of choice, and the patient should be helped to come to the correct decision on an individual basis.

Pre-operative assessment (see Ch. 2)

Range of movement of shoulder girdle, shoulder joint, elbow, pronation and supination, and wrist movement.

Muscle power controlling these joints. If a patient has no active elbow flexion, an above-elbow amputation will be required; if no active shoulder movement is possible, a shoulder arthrodesis may be indicated.

Pain control. Experience has shown that there is a link between pain in the arm in the pre-amputation phase and phantom pain occurring postoperatively; therefore pain relief prior to amputation is essential. However, amputation should not be performed in order to relieve pain: other treatment modalities should be explored.

Scar tissue. If a patient has extensive surgical or burn scars, the condition of the skin may dictate the level of amputation both for healing of the stump and for subsequent limb fitting.

Psychological aspects of amputation

Whatever the cause of the amputation, the loss of an arm has serious psychological implications. The upper limb, and in particular the hand, play an important part in self-image, in personality development and in manipulative skills. As stated by Crossthwaite Eyre (1979):

Arms and particularly hands are an integral part of personality development and are an extremely complex mechanical part of our bodies. They are a means of expression of self through affection, sexual identity, manual dexterity, sometimes speech and importantly as a means of providing for the family as tools of work. Very often the initial shock of losing an upper limb affects the patient's attitude towards his total body image, subjecting him to feelings of inadequacy and incapacity. These factors are augmented when the dominant side is affected. The realisation that present technology is so far unable to provide a replacement with perfect or near-perfect function, or sensation, and can offer only a partial degree of cosmetic acceptability, causes additional concern. Therefore these individuals need a great deal of psychological support and encouragement which must continue until they return to their normal lifestyle.

This psychological disturbance after limb loss must be handled sensitively and realistically. It is frequently the therapists within the multi-disciplinary team who can provide much of the help that is required, reassuring the amputee by planning treatment programmes directed towards ultimate independence with or without the use of a prosthesis. Knowledge of what can be achieved is important at this stage to give the patient a realistic view of the future.

Hand dominance

Loss of the dominant hand is a factor requiring special attention. Upper limb prostheses do not provide sensory feedback, although some bio-feedback is provided in working the conventional body-powered limb. (This feedback is mainly related to an awareness of the power required to work a terminal device.) It is, therefore, very important to encourage patients to develop competence in the use of the non-dominant hand, so that they can become skilled in fine dexterity where sensory input is essential. This must commence from the first postoperative day and will be of great advantage when the prosthesis is fitted and prosthetic rehabilitation commences.

Any activity to give the amputee practice with the non-dominant hand should be encouraged in order to develop manipulative skills. The amputee should be encouraged to dress and feed himself but consideration must be given to the level of frustration that is tolerable.

Some amputees can achieve adequate writing skills with a prosthesis, but the majority will, eventually, write better with the remaining hand; therefore practice should start as soon as possible. The bilateral arm amputee will probably write better with the longer stump, not necessarily the dominant arm. All possibilities should be encouraged.

Learning to write again must be presented like a child learning, starting with an easy pen such as a fibre-tip. Scribbling exercises should be begun initially rather than writing letters. This encourages a relaxed grip on the pen and will result in better writing in future.

Pre-prosthetic treatment

The aims of treatment are:
— Joint mobility and muscle strength
— Control of oedema
— Functional movement
— Desensitising the stump
— Psychological adaptation.

Joint mobility and muscle strength

Early active movements of all joints above the level of amputation, including the whole of the shoulder girdle and neck, should be commenced with the physiotherapist on the first postoperative day. Resisted active exercises can commence as pain permits.

These exercises should concentrate particularly on all movements of the shoulder joint and shoulder girdle. Ability to retain the smooth gliding movement of the scapula on the chest wall in protraction is essential. This movement, coupled with flexion of the shoulder joint, is the main power force for working a body-powered prosthesis, particularly for the above-elbow amputee. The shoulder joint can be exercised with

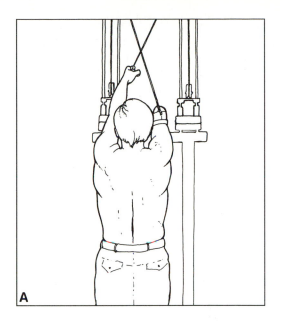

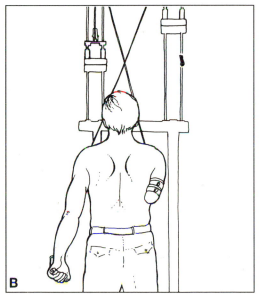

Fig. 17.1 An above-elbow amputee mobilising and strengthening the shoulder girdle and shoulder joint, using a Westminster pulley system. Note the scapular excursion between (A) and (B).

manually resisted techniques, such as proprioceptive neuromuscular facilitation, or by the use of a pulley system (Fig. 17.1). Bilateral activities are particularly useful.

If the elbow joint is present, a full range of

movement must be achieved daily to prevent any flexion contractures. The forearm support prone position is useful for performing resisted head and neck patterns. This encourages shoulder girdle movement and biceps and triceps activity, as well as accustoming the stump to pressure.

The general posture of the neck and upper trunk must be corrected and trunk rotation during walking must be maintained. Single arm amputees tend to flex towards the affected side. The trunk may become rather rigid during walking, as loss of arm swing and trunk rotation may lead to a feeling of imbalance. Retraining of postural reactions, by use of manually resisted

exercises and wobble boards, either in lying, sitting or standing, must start early in the exercise programme. The arm amputee must also be encouraged to try different paces of gait, i.e. jogging, running, etc., as these activities will initially feel very different.

As with lower extremity amputees, sport and leisure pursuits must be explored later on, once rehabilitation is near completion.

Control of oedema

Elevation of the upper limb stump is difficult to achieve. Some find a sling in bed helpful so the

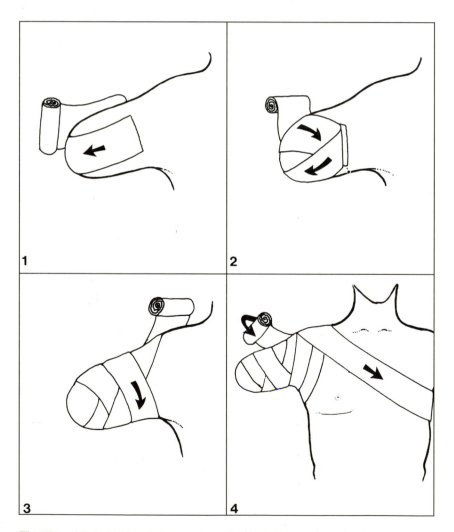

Fig. 17.2 Method of bandaging an above-elbow stump.

stump is elevated at night. Some below-elbow amputees may find a sling helpful during the day but care must be taken that the elbow does not become flexed and the shoulder internally rotated.

Active contraction of the stump muscles should be encouraged at regular intervals. General use of the stump in everyday activity will help reduce oedema.

Stump bandaging may be commenced once the wound is healed and sutures are removed (see Fig. 17.2). The aim is to control oedema and condition the stump to prosthetic wear. Care should be taken to ensure that the joints above the level of amputation can move freely and that pressure is exerted on the distal end of the stump with diagonal turns. A badly applied bandage is worse than no bandage; at no time should a tourniquet effect be attained. These principles are the same as for the lower limb amputees (see Ch. 3). Pressure garments may also be used, giving a more consistent degree of pressure.

Functional movement

In order to maintain these movement patterns, use of the stump should be encouraged as soon as possible. Frequently, the occupational therapist will be involved at this stage.

A simple leather gauntlet (Fig. 17.3) can be applied over the dressing to which simple devices can be attached, and the amputee is encouraged to carry out tasks using the stump. Care must be taken to keep these activities realistic and practical. This is more easily achieved with a below-elbow amputee. A fork can be attached as a pusher for bilateral feeding, and is used with a spoon in the remaining hand. Typing with a simple peg attached to the gauntlet helps retrain proprioception. Painting with a paint brush at an easel or on a table encourages control of the stump in finer precision activity; in addition, it helps to develop control in differing shoulder girdle ranges of movement.

Because of very unequal arm lengths, activities for the above-elbow amputee are more difficult to plan. However, an extended table-tennis bat attached to the gauntlet with a figure-of-eight strap around the opposite axilla can be used to encourage forward shoulder flexion (Fig. 17.4).

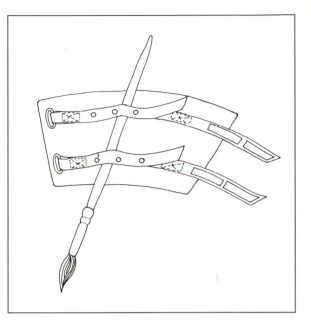

Fig. 17.3 A pre-prosthetic leather gauntlet, with paintbrush attached. (Reproduced by kind permission of Baillière Tindall, from Robertson E. 1978 Rehabilitation of arm amputees and limb deficient children.)

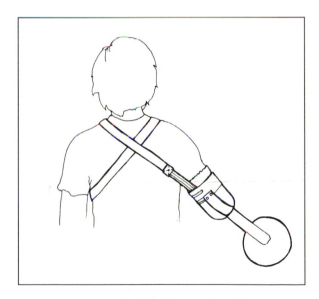

Fig. 17.4 A pre-prosthetic leather gauntlet, with extended table-tennis bat attached. (Reproduced by kind permission of Baillière Tindall, from Robertson E. 1978 Rehabilitation of arm amputees and limb deficient children.)

Desensitising the stump

The amputee should be encouraged to handle the stump as soon as possible, starting with gentle massage over the dressing, progressing to more aggressive movement and percussion. The ability to reach directly to the end of the stump with the remaining hand should be achievable by the second week. When the stump is healed, massage with hydrous wool fat cream or other non-allergic moisturising cream is encouraged to condition the skin, prevent adhesions and continue to desensitise the stump.

If the amputee is not willing to handle the stump it may become hypersensitive and the amputee becomes very protective of it. This is a difficult cycle to break and involves handling the stump for 5 minutes once an hour using percussion techniques within the amputee's tolerance.

The amputee's partner/parent/carer should also be encouraged to look at and handle the stump. They may find this very difficult initially. Discussion about phantom sensation should be open and honest. Most amputees find that the sensation changes over a period of time; for many it eventually goes, but some will find the phantom sensation remains.

Psychological adaptation

Amputees need to be allowed to grieve the loss of the limb. Often they will progress through a normal grief pattern. The attitude of staff and the amputee's friends and relatives is important in the early days post-amputation. Some amputees require the help of specific professional counselling to enable them to adapt satisfactorily to their new situation. The families of amputees may also require help adjusting to the change in circumstances.

Immediate postoperative fitting

Immediate postoperative fitting came into vogue for lower-limb amputees in the 1960s; it did not achieve great success in the UK because of the problems of poor vascularity and healing. It still has a place for upper limb amputees, if the whole team of surgeon, therapists, consultant in rehabilitation and prosthetist is on site to constantly monitor the fit and the use of the limb.

Where this technique is used, a temporary prosthesis is fitted either in the operating theatre or during the first few days postoperatively. For below-elbow amputees, the socket is made of a thermoplastic material or plaster-of-Paris. A woollen sock is incorporated into the socket. A wrist unit and straps are fitted. Thus within 2–3 days the patient has a functional artificial limb. As the stump reduces in size more stump socks are worn. This system is used very rarely for above-elbow amputees, but a redundant above-elbow prosthesis can be used, the socket split and Velcro straps fixed circumferentially in order to allow for changes in the size of the stump. An inner lining of Plastazote or Velvetex is supplied.

Advantages

The advantages of immediate postoperative fitting for upper limb amputees are as follows:

— *Psychological improvement*: the patient immediately uses the prosthesis and is made aware of its potential.
— *Control of oedema*: this is achieved by the encasement of the stump in a socket.
— *Neurophysiological movement patterns* are retained by immediate use of the stump in the prosthesis.
— *Active movements*: patterns of movement associated with the use of the prosthesis, in particular, are performed. However, in the early stages it is also necessary to perform an active exercise programme without the prosthesis (see p. 193).
— *Training in the use of the prosthesis*: this commences much earlier and makes final re-education with the definitive prosthesis more effective.

It must be stressed that the immediate postoperative fitting technique should only be used where the medical, therapeutic and prosthetic skills required are available. Without the full team being available, any attempts to carry out this technique could be harmful rather than beneficial to the amputee.

Levels of amputation and prostheses

There are optimal levels of amputation in the upper limb as with lower limb. For all active amputees these optimal levels should, as far as possible, be chosen. Preservation of length of stump is advantageous in order to act as a lever, but the stump should be short enough to allow for prosthetic components, such as wrist or elbow unit, to be fitted, thus enabling a functional and cosmetic artificial replacement to be supplied.

Upper limb prostheses may be cosmetic, or functional, or a combination of both. The stump length and the functional/cosmetic requirements need to be taken into account when discussing prostheses. An amputee may initially require a cosmetic prosthesis, but after a period of adjustment find more function is required. An amputee working in heavy industry may require a prosthesis that is very robust and cosmesis is of less importance than strength and function. It is important to assess and reassess the amputees' needs regularly.

The socket may be made of leather, plastic, or plastic lined with either leather or silicone. The function may be through body power or external power, or the arm may be purely cosmetic.

Forequarter amputation

This is usually performed for malignant disease around the shoulder joint. It involves the removal of the clavicle and scapula as well as the whole arm, and leaves the patient with a gross disfigurement. Initially, the need is for cosmesis, and a light shoulder cap that will not cause pressure on the chest wall but allows clothing to be worn to give a normal outline should be fitted postoperatively (Fig. 17.5). Early referral to the DSC is essential to supply this shoulder cap, which is both for cosmetic replacement and protection. Many patients opt to wear this device definitively. A prosthesis may be supplied and it is made of light foam with a simple elbow and a cosmetic hand. A functional prosthesis is usually too heavy to be tolerated. However, patients who have a broad back may manage an electrically powered prosthesis where the heavy weight is tolerated because of the function.

Shoulder disarticulation

This is also referred to as a through-shoulder amputation. The clavicle and acromion process should be trimmed to leave a rounded contour in order to prevent the protuberance causing discomfort when a socket is fitted.

The working prosthesis is similar to an above-elbow prosthesis but requires an extended shoulder cap in order to give additional contour and fixing points for harnessing. The limb incorporates an elbow mechanism for active flexion

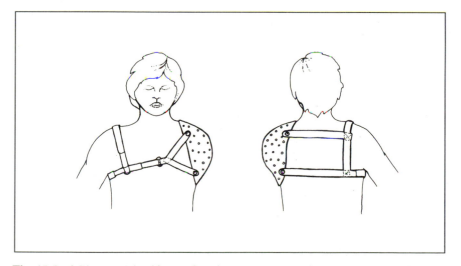

Fig. 17.5 A Plastazote shoulder cap for a forequarter amputation.

which is achieved by protraction of the shoulder girdle.

The elbow mechanism is locked and unlocked by the remaining hand. The functional benefits of the prosthesis are limited and the prosthesis is used more as a steadying device for holding down objects whilst the amputee is writing or cutting, etc.

Electrically powered devices are more easy to operate and therefore the prosthesis is more functional. However, such prostheses are heavy and can generally only be tolerated by broad-backed, healthy amputees. A very mobile shoulder girdle and remaining shoulder joint are essential for successful operation of the terminal device.

Above-elbow

The optimum site for an above-elbow amputation is 10 cm above the elbow joint, measured from the olecranon. This allows space for the elbow mechanism of the prosthesis to fit into the humeral section, and ensure that the prosthesis elbow joint is at the anatomical level. Additionally, it provides a good length of stump for leverage and prosthetic control. A stump shorter than 4 cm measured from the anterior axillary fold of the shoulder is considered prosthetically in the same way as for a shoulder disarticulation.

An above-elbow prosthesis incorporates harnessing to hold the prosthesis in position and to allow the patient to activate it (see Fig. 17.6).

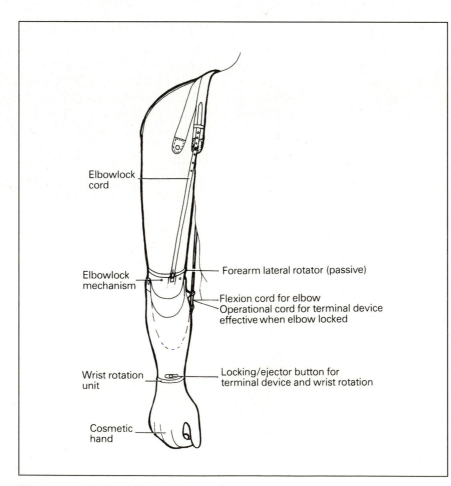

Fig. 17.6   An above-elbow prosthesis.

The elbow joint is flexed by humeral flexion and shoulder girdle protraction, putting tension on the operating cord (see Fig. 17.7). To lock the elbow in the desired position the patient either pulls the locking strap with his remaining hand or uses the automatic locking mechanism. The latter is to be encouraged if it is possible, as it allows the remaining hand freedom. The mechanism is operated by a movement of the shoulder joint which pulls on the lock cord: shoulder depression, extension, internal rotation and abduction, or 'nudging someone in the ribs'. The same movement is required to unlock the elbow. An amputee with a very short stump or with brachial plexus damage will rarely achieve this movement and will operate the lock with the remaining hand. A hand-operated elbow unit, i.e. a switch on the forearm, rather than the strap, may be considered. This is a lighter unit, but has fewer locking positions.

To compensate for loss of internal and external rotation at the shoulder joint and yet allow the patient the opportunity to position the forearm in a good working position, a mechanism is incorporated in the lower end of the humeral section immediately above the elbow joint. This mechanism is a friction joint, passively rotated with the amputee's remaining hand in order to place the forearm in the desired position. It can be locked by a simple push button.

The wrist unit, allowing rotation through 360° of any terminal device being worn, has a push-button mechanism to enable removal or locking of the device. Once the elbow is locked, the movements and power used for elbow flexion are transmitted via the operating cord to the terminal device which is then activated.

Elbow disarticulation

This level of amputation has the disadvantage that the elbow mechanism now has to be fitted externally. There is no rotation unit at the elbow. Functionally, this level of amputation has no advantage over the optimum above-elbow level. However, there may be situations where this is the optimum level of amputation for a particular patient, e.g. bilateral amputee or a non-limb wearer.

Below-elbow

The optimum amputation level for fitting a below-elbow prosthesis is 8 cm above the ulnar styloid to allow room for the wrist unit and maintain the same length on the remaining arm.

The socket can be of two types:

1. A cup socket held on by a harness which incorporates the operating cord, allowing the

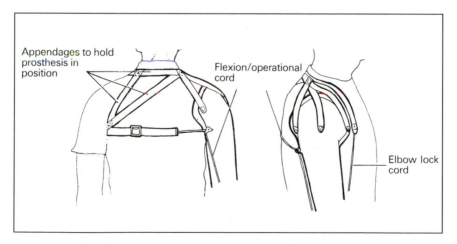

Fig. 17.7   A suspension system for an above-elbow prosthesis.

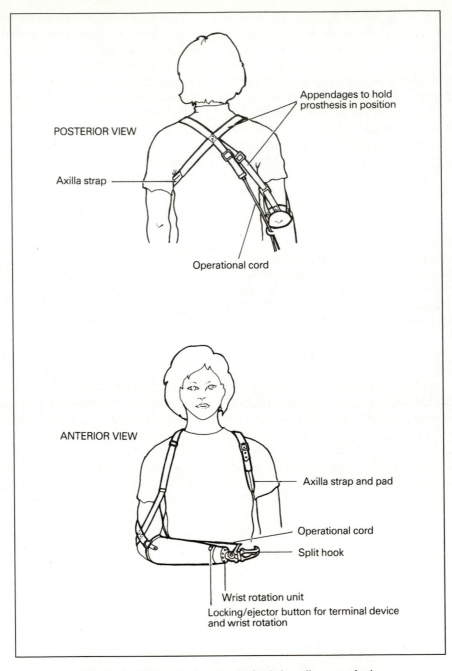

POSTERIOR VIEW

Appendages to hold
prosthesis in position

Axilla strap

Operational cord

ANTERIOR VIEW

Axilla strap and pad

Operational cord

Split hook

Wrist rotation unit
Locking/ejector button for terminal device
and wrist rotation

Fig. 17.8 Suspension for a cup socket below-elbow prosthesis.

patient to activate the terminal device (Fig. 17.8). This socket is used for:

— new amputees, as their stump is still reducing in size
— amputees who require the prosthesis to carry heavy weights, as the weight is therefore distributed across their shoulders
— amputees with very short stumps, when a self-suspending socket may be very difficult to fit.

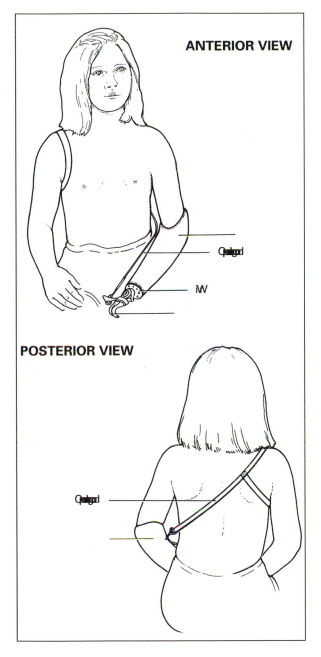

Fig. 17.9 Supracondular self-suspending socket for a below-elbow prosthesis.

2. A self-suspending/supracondylar socket (Fig. 17.9) in which the operating cord is on a loop harness which activates the terminal device. This can be removed when the prosthesis is worn as a cosmetic device only.

The wrist unit is the same as in the above elbow prosthesis. The device is operated by elbow extension and shoulder flexion and/or shoulder girdle protraction (see p. 197).

Wrist disarticulation

The prosthesis is sometimes made with a split forearm piece, enabling the amputee to utilise the remaining functions of pronation and supination. The prosthesis is likely to be longer than the remaining arm and may be bulbous at the distal end.

Partial hand

Cosmetic and functional devices are available for varying types of amputation, but they always have to be considered on an individual basis. The available function should be assessed without hardware initially; therapy may be required to improve function. If a functional device is required it is often designed by the prosthetist following discussion with the amputee, occupational therapist and doctor. Devices are most often required for specific tasks and a device can also be supplied for cosmetic purposes.

Terminal devices

Prostheses can be supplied with a *cosmetic hand*, the fingers of which can be moved passively; they have limited functional value, but are the best cosmetic replacements.

A *mechanical hand* is available where index and middle fingers form a three-point grip against the thumb. The hand is opened by tension on the operating cord pulling the thumb and fingers apart. This hand can serve a purpose for amputees not demanding a high level of manipulative skill from the prosthesis. This is determined by the amputee's lifestyle and employment requirements.

The most commonly used terminal device is the *split hook*, which allows a high degree of manipulative skill (see Fig. 17.10). It has one fixed and one movable jaw, the latter being activated by body power. It is opened actively, and closes passively once tension is released. The grip power is determined by strong rubber bands,

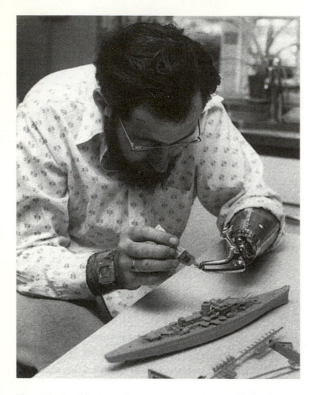

Fig. 17.10   A below-elbow amputee using a split hook with a high degree of manipulative skill. (Reproduced by kind permission of Baillière Tindall, from Robertson E 1978 Rehabilitation of arm amputees and limb deficient children.)

against which force the body power has to work to open the jaw. The greater the pinch grip required, the stronger the resistance of the bands needs to be, and consequently greater body power is required to open it. This accounts for the need to strengthen the amputee's shoulder girdle muscles throughout the pre-prosthetic phase. The length of stump, coupled with shoulder girdle power, will determine the amount of grip that can be achieved.

There are additional terminal devices which can be supplied for specific tasks, and amputees are assessed for these during the prosthetic rehabilitation period.

Prosthetic rehabilitation with body-powered prostheses

A programme of prosthetic rehabilitation should be initiated immediately the patient has taken delivery of the prosthesis. Prosthetic rehabilitation is provided by the occupational therapy service, either in a hospital department associated with a DSC, or in a specialised unit within the DSC.

It is important that the advantages of prosthetic rehabilitation are made known to the amputee early on, for without it the prosthesis can easily become a 'sleeve filler' with only limited functional use.

Initially, control of the prosthesis will be taught but, once this is achieved, bimanual activities will be introduced. Guided by the occupational therapist, the amputee learns to use the prosthesis in an automatic way to acquire the skills required for his normal lifestyle.

Training for a below-elbow amputee generally requires three to four sessions and for an above-elbow amputee five to six sessions. This may take the form of several consecutive days or separate days. It is helpful to consolidate and perfect the skills that have been learned and acquired in the normal routine of everyday life. These skills can be increased and improved on as training progresses. Amputees with additional disabilities will require more training. Psychological rehabilitation may take considerably longer than prosthetic training.

Procedure of prosthetic rehabilitation

The procedure of prosthetic education for the single arm amputee must incorporate the following:

1. Checking the fit of the prosthesis
2. Understanding the working parts of the prosthesis
3. Application of the prosthesis
4. Personal independence training
5. Prosthetic training
6. Use of terminal devices.

1. Checking the fit of the prosthesis

The prosthetist will have carried out this procedure at the time of delivery. However, it is essential that the occupational therapist also examines the fit, as immediate use of the prosthesis in activity can require minor adjustment, to ensure that the amputee is acquiring maximum response from all shoulder girdle movement. As little as 1 cm of slack in the operating cords can cause unnecessary effort on the part of the amputee in order to flex the elbow or work the terminal device.

2. Understanding the working parts of the prosthesis

Because of the wide range of working parts incorporated in an upper limb prosthesis, the amputee must have time to 'play' with it and understand how it works. There may be advantages in carrying out this exercise initially with another prosthesis as a table model. Once the amputee is familiar with the hardware, confidence in its potential use can be achieved.

3. Application of the prosthesis

The patient must learn how to put on and take off the prosthesis. Most single arm amputees find that this presents few problems, and once the technique has been grasped, practice will make it a routine activity. A stump sock may be worn. The harness may be worn over a vest. The opposite axilla pad can cause tenderness initially and personal hygiene of this area is essential. The skin will toughen in time and it is not helpful to place additional padding under this strap. For the below-elbow amputee with a cup socket and harness, positioning the stump between the straps has to be mastered in order that the straps may lie in the correct position once the prosthesis is on. For above-elbow amputees there are several ways of donning and doffing the prosthesis depending on the length of stump and preference of the amputee.

4. Personal independence training

Activities of daily living, for single arm amputees, rarely present problems unless there are additional disabilities. Dressing, once the prosthesis has been applied, is carried out mainly as a one-handed activity, although a terminal device, such as a split hook, can be useful as a grasping, stabilising

tool when the amputee is doing up a tie or pulling up a zip. Washing and bathing are undertaken without the prosthesis.

Managing cutlery is taught so that the amputee can become independent in feeding. It is easier for the amputee to hold the knife in the prosthesis, taking food to the mouth with the remaining hand.

5. Prosthetic training

The objective here is to identify the particular needs of the individual and plan a treatment programme with graded activity in order to achieve that end. Each individual requires specific manipulative skills according to their work and leisure interests. If possible, these skills must be included in the rehabilitation programme. A hospital department may not be able to provide training in all of these, but simulated activities which require the same type of coordinated movement and skill can be used. Amputees, with guidance from the occupational therapist, can then adapt these skills to their personal situation in the normal work and home environment.

The first task for the amputee is to gain control of the terminal device, and the most effective way of doing this is with the split hook. Repeated opening and closing to grasp objects is practised, and all types of peg-board games with varying sizes of pegs are ideal for this. Computer games can be used to retrain 'hand'/eye coordination.

Once the amputee has begun to gain control of the prosthesis, bimanual activities are introduced; this can be done on the first day, beginning with simple tasks and progressing to the more complex. Clerical tasks, domestic work, constructional models, carpentry, gardening are all possibilities, but selection of activities by the occupational therapist is of great importance as patients may become frustrated if unable to do a task satisfactorily. Driving a car, sewing, knitting, golf, cricket, billiards, fishing — there is no limit of the number of leisure pursuits that can be tried out. The amputee should be shown ways of achieving these activities so that practice can be continued at home.

Many arm amputees will return to their former employment, either working at the same job or working in a different capacity with the same employer. However, some may require specific vocational retraining following their initial prosthetic rehabilitation; these patients should be advised to contact the disablement resettlement officer at their local Job Centre.

6. Use of terminal devices

For the majority of amputees the split hook will prove to be the most universally effective tool. Cosmetically it does not have great appeal and the patient may have to experience its effectiveness before accepting it. There are other terminal devices for specific tasks such as a spade grip for gardening and a universal toolholder for mechanical work. Should an amputee have a work situation or leisure interest that calls for a special device to be designed, the research and development team of the prosthetic manufacturers, in collaboration with the occupational therapist, may be able to make a one-off device.

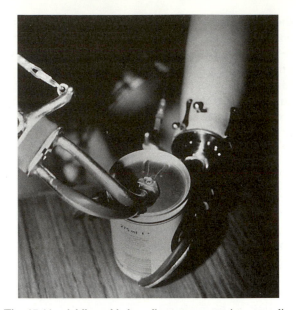

Fig. 17.11   A bilateral below elbow amputee using two split hooks to open a ring-pull can. (Photograph by kind permission of the Medical Photography Department, Queen Mary's University Hospital, Roehampton.)

BILATERAL ARM AMPUTEES

To lose one arm is a traumatic experience. For a patient to lose both arms is a tragedy. Bilateral arm amputees due to acquired amputation are fortunately very small in number; there are about two patients a year in the UK.

However, because of the severity of the disability, very sensitive care must be given in the early stages of treatment. The pre-prosthetic programme should include all the objectives listed above for the single arm amputee. When ready — physically and psychologically — for prosthetic management, the bilateral arm amputee should attend a specialised occupational therapy department where there are the facilities and expertise for effective prosthetic rehabilitation. Most bilateral arm amputees, once they appreciate the functional possibilities that prostheses can offer them, are highly motivated towards success, as this is their only hope of independence (see Fig. 17.11).

Prosthetic rehabilitation concentrates in the first instance on personal independence in feeding, toileting, dressing and communication skills. Concentrated repetitive practice is required, with direction and guidance being given by the occupational therapist, who must counsel, encourage and set realistic goals for achievement so that the amputee's expectations are not shattered. Once the amputee has acquired some independence (this may take 3–6 weeks), a period at home to consolidate the skills should be planned. A further period of concentrated treatment to incorporate work activities and leisure pursuits is best tackled separately, if possible as phase two of the programme; this may last a further 2–4 weeks.

It can be helpful for the new amputee to meet an established bilateral arm amputee, who has adapted to life with two artificial arms and managed to assume a useful and acceptable lifestyle. This introduction must be carefully timed and planned, and is best left to the staff who are employed at the centre where prosthetic rehabilitation is to be carried out and who understand the finer points of management of such a patient.

CONGENITAL LIMB DEFICIENCY

It is a great shock to parents when a child is born with part of a limb missing. This is a very rare occurrence; some parents (and indeed occasionally the medical staff) have never heard of such an event before and therefore believe that they and their child are unique and that no-one will be able to help them or understand their problem.

The most common forms of congenital deficiency occur in the upper limbs, although deficiencies of the lower limbs are also seen. The ratio of upper to lower limb defects in this group of patients is about 5 : 1.

In 1978 the Association for Children with Hand and Arm Deficiency (REACH) was formed. They bring together parents of children with upper limb deficiencies through a national and regional network. They produce a newsletter and helpful leaflets giving early advice to parents. Therapists who know of any child born with upper limb deficiency, through working in an obstetric unit or paediatric department, should encourage the family to contact REACH as soon as possible. This should be followed by early referral to their local DSC, ideally when the child is 4–6 weeks old. At this stage, the baby is assessed, but the visit is primarily for the parents. It is an opportunity to meet the rehabilitation consultant and occupational therapist, to answer the parents' questions, to discuss the child's prosthetic management and to see some of the prosthetic options available. It may also be an opportunity to meet a similar family.

Although all DSCs can deal with the simpler deficiencies, any child with complex deficiencies should be referred to a specialist centre, such as these at Roehampton, Manchester or Edinburgh, where expertise in management is available.

The most common upper limb deficiency is the absence of a hand and lower third of the forearm; this is known as a terminal transverse arrest. The ratio of incidence in males to females is 1 : 1; the ratio of incidence of left to right is 2 : 1, but the reason for this is unknown (see Ch. 2).

When treating children with any form of deficiency it is important that the therapist sees them in the context of the family since the parents are co-therapists, carrying out treatment regimes at home. Their ability to do this will depend on the advice and guidance given to them by the occupational therapist. Siblings will also play their part and it may be helpful for them to attend one or two of the training sessions.

Prosthetic management

The optimal time for fitting a young child with an upper limb prosthesis has been heavily debated; the current view leans towards an early fitting. It is therefore normal practice to fit a child with a cosmetic arm at 5–6 months. This is the time when a child is beginning to sit independently. The prosthesis enables the child to become used to having a full length arm, so 'hand'/eye coordination is correctly formulated, and the child becomes accustomed to wearing a prosthesis. Some parents find the concern and comments of the public hard to come to terms with; the presence of the cosmetic hand at the end of the sleeve makes the disability less obvious (see Fig. 17.12).

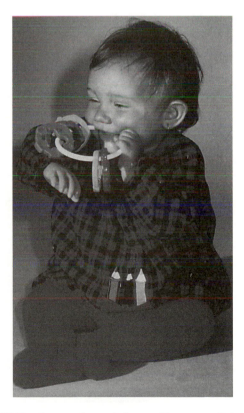

Fig. 17.12 A cosmetic arm being used by a young baby for bilateral activity play. (Photograph by kind permission of J. C. Lamparter and the Medical Photography Department, Queen Mary's University Hospital, Roehampton.)

The prosthesis can be used as a stabilising device, for hitting mobiles and towers, for holding large toys in a bimanual grasp. The prosthesis has to be replaced at regular intervals as the child grows.

At 18 months, when the child is walking securely and beginning to be interested in manipulative skills the child is fitted with its first functional limb. This may be the infant split hook or the Canadian Amputee Prosthetic Project (CAPP) device, more like a crab's claw. There are advantages and disadvantages of each and the child needs to be assessed as an individual and the parents' views sought.

Training of the child and parents begins when the first functional prosthesis is collected and should consist of several short sessions as the child's concentration span at this age is very limited. Play activities will be used and must be matched to the normal developmental milestones of the child and the type of toys currently available. Many of the educational-type toys are useful as specific treatment media in structured sessions, but free play activity must also be allowed in order to let the child experiment.

Regular review every 3 months is the most beneficial way of charting progress. A treatment session with the occupational therapist should be time-tabled into these routine visits to the DSC to identify any difficulties or increase the range of activities undertaken. A constant check will be kept on the need to increase the size of the prosthesis as the child grows.

At 3–3.5 years, the child is considered for a myoelectric prosthesis (see Fig. 17.13). Assessment takes into consideration:

— The child's maturity
— The child's ability to dissociate contractions of wrist flexors and extensors
— Hand size
— Previous limb wearing.

When the timing is considered appropriate by the doctor, occupational therapist, prosthetist and parents, a cast is taken and a training programme

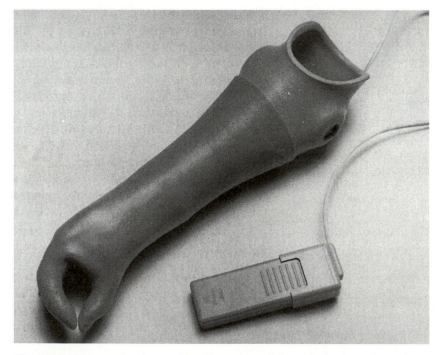

Fig. 17.13 The myoelectric arm. Mounting point and electrode are situated over the forearm flexors. A 6 volt battery and lead and cosmetic glove are shown. The hand is closed in a three-point grip. (Photograph reproduced by kind permission of Hugh Steeper & Co. Ltd.)

arranged. If possible this should be on 3 consecutive days.

Training takes a similar form to previous sessions: unilateral activities, e.g. puzzles, to learn hand control, and bilateral activities of an appropriate level for the child, e.g. cutting, threading, construction toys (see Fig. 17.14).

During this training period, the fit of the socket should be checked, and care of the prosthesis discussed with the parent. If the child is attending nursery, the staff should be contacted and given information about the prosthesis.

As the child approaches school age, the parents may need advice in how to introduce their child to a classroom situation. Most children with upper limb deficiencies attend normal school, and it can be helpful, if the parents are in agreement, for the occupational therapist to carry out a school visit and advise the teacher on how to accept and make the most of the child's potential.

Children's needs change dramatically as they grow. A constant dialogue must be maintained between the occupational therapist and family to ascertain that these needs are being recognised and catered for, and if necessary further training may be arranged. This will increase the range of activities available to the child and will follow the type of bimanual approach used for adult amputees.

There may be phases when the child will reject the prosthesis and these should be recognised and accepted. Often these periods are short but the child must be allowed to decide when to return to prosthetic use.

Children continue to attend a DSC for review on a regular basis up to adulthood, then yearly attendances may be all that is needed. By then they should have acquired all the skills necessary to live a normal life with the means of choosing a career and lifestyle that will not be hampered by their limb deficiency.

EXTERNALLY POWERED PROSTHESES

History of external power

Myoelectric hands for below-elbow adult amputees in the UK were experimented with in the 1950s without much success. They were heavy, mechanically unreliable and slow to open and close. Amputees who were fitted with these soon rejected them and returned to body-powered prostheses. During the thalidomide tragedy in 1960, another type of external power was utilised in the form of a compressed carbon dioxide gas cylinder carried on the child. The gas powered the opening and closing of a small split hook, and in some cases a wrist rotation unit. The amount of hardware the child had to wear for the small return in function finally led to its rejection.

In the USA, Canada and Germany, work went on to develop electrically powered hands for adults, and these programmes continued, with Italy joining at a later date. A limited amount of the development was for children.

In the early 1970s, a mechanical hand, powered electrically by muscle contraction, was developed for young children in Sweden. This created international interest and the Department of Health introduced it into the UK in 1979. A research

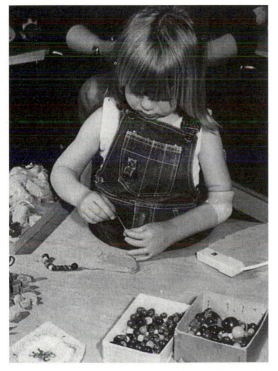

Fig. 17.14 A congenital below-elbow child amputee using a myoelectric arm. During a free-play activity session in the Arm Training Unit, her mother is present as a co-therapist.

project lasting 3 years was planned in order to evaluate its effectiveness for children aged 3.5–4.5 years.

The research showed that children within this age group could make good use of the hand, parents were pleased with it and preferred it to a body-powered limb. As a result of this project, the myoelectric prosthesis for below-elbow amputees became available on prescription. Larger hand sizes were developed and now the myoelectric hand is available to all amputees and limb deficient children over the age of 3 years.

Types of prosthesis

There are two main types of electrically powered prostheses: myoelectric and those utilising a servo system.

Myoelectric

The myoelectric prosthesis has a supracondylar self-suspending socket in which two electrodes are mounted over the wrist flexor and extensor muscle bulks of the forearm. On contraction of the wrist flexors the electric impulse is picked up by the medial electrode, releasing power from the 6 volt battery situated in the forearm. This power is transmitted to the motor in the hand which causes the hand to close. When the wrist extensors contract this causes the hand to open. The main advantages of this device are the combination of function with cosmesis and the ability to use the hand in any range of elbow or shoulder position, e.g. up above the head. This contrasts with the split hook, where opening and closing depends on shoulder flexion and elbow extension, thus only permitting active use below shoulder height and in front of the body. In addition, a harness is not needed for the myoelectric device. It must be stressed, however, that the functional use of the hand is not as precise as the split hook, but it does allow for a constant, more powerful grip. It is not possible at present to interchange an electric hand with other terminal devices such as the split hook. There are a few above-elbow amputees who are able to operate myoelectric controls using biceps and triceps.

The prosthesis would probably have a body-powered automatic elbow unit.

Servo mechanisms

Many above-elbow amputees are not able to achieve myoelectric control and for them a servo system may be more appropriate. This is similar to the body-powered prosthesis but only 1 cm of shoulder protraction is required to fully open the hand. This enables the amputee to have a cosmetic hand and a strong grip. The hand can also be operated by shoulder elevation using a strap to a waist belt.

Some below-elbow amputees may benefit from this system if they cannot use myoelectric controls, e.g. if they have excessive scarring which may not allow the electrical impulses to be picked up by the electrodes, or the stump is very short.

Rehabilitation with externally powered prostheses

Amputees may be considered for an electrically powered prosthesis from 6 months postamputation. By this stage they are accustomed to wearing a prosthesis, have become used to the weight and any oedema should have subsided. It is essential that the socket, especially for the myoelectric prosthesis, is close-fitting. It is important that the amputee is well adjusted to the amputation and is realistic about the potential of the electric prosthesis.

Training

Training with electric prostheses follows similar lines to that for body-powered prostheses.

1. Checking the fit

The patient needs to wear and use the prosthesis for 15–20 minutes before checking the fit; there should be clear, but not 'angry', marks on the stump where the electrodes are sited. The occupational therapist should liaise with the prosthetist to enable alterations to the fit of the socket to be carried out during rehabilitation.

2. Understanding the working parts of the prosthesis

The method of operation of the hand should be explained to the amputee in an appropriate manner. There is a friction wrist, and maybe an on/off switch, allowing power to the hand to be switched off. The hands for adults have a thumb break, enabling a grip release, e.g. when the battery has run out. The charging of the battery and use of the battery charger, care of the cosmetic glove and how to change the glove if it becomes damaged must be explained. The hand must not be immersed in water.

3. Personal independence training

Donning and doffing the prosthesis must be practised. Some skills are now easier for the patient to achieve, e.g. tying a shoe lace, as now the hand can be closed when the elbow is in extension.

4. Prosthetic training

As with the body-powered prosthesis this will start with unilateral exercises, concentrating initially on hand control. Adjustments to the electrode sensitivity settings, or to the operational cord for the servo hand, may be required. Training will progress from unilateral to bilateral exercise.

5. Terminal devices

At present it is not possible to remove the electric hand from the forearm. Work is being carried out on a wrist disconnector so that the hand can be removed and any terminal device fitted in its place. Tweezers and a cup for holding a driving knob of a car can be held in the hand.

It is important to remember that electric power will not revolutionise the future for all arm amputees; for some patients, body power will be the most effective. The needs and preferences of the individual amputee should always be remembered when considering the value of body power versus electric power.

PROSTHESES INFORMATION

Detailed information regarding prostheses available in the UK can be obtained from manufacturers. The addresses are listed in the Appendix.

REFERENCES

Angliss V 1981 Early referral to limb deficiency clinics. Prosthetics and Orthotics International 5: 141–143
Bhala R P, Schultz C F 1982 Golf club holder for upper-extremity amputee golfers. Archives of Physical Medicine and Rehabilitation 63: 339–341
Crosthwaite Eyre N 1979 Rehabilitation of the upper limb amputee. Physiotherapy 65(1): 9–12
Curran B, Hambrey R 1991 The prosthetic treatment of upper limb deficiency. Prosthetics and Orthotics International 15: 82–87
Enzinna A J 1975 Orientation and mobility for a totally blind bilateral hand amputee. New Outlook March: 103–108
Hambrey R, Withinshaw G 1990 Electrically powered upper limb prostheses: their development and application. British Journal of Occupational Therapy 53(1): 7–11
Hermansson L M 1991 Structured training of children fitted with myoelectric prostheses. Prosthetics and Orthotics International 15: 88–92
Hughes S 1980 Abnormalities of the limbs. Nursing Mirror 16 October: 17–20
Kulkarni J 1990 Partial hand prostheses: a clinical profile. British Journal of Occupational Therapy 53(5): 200–201
Malone J M, Fleming L L, Roberson J, Whitesides T E, Leal J M, Poole J U, Sternstein Grodin R 1984 Immediate, early and late postsurgical management of upper-limb amputation. Journal of Rehabilitation Research and Development 21(1): 33–41
Marquardt E G 1983 A holistic approach to rehabilitation for the limb-deficient child. Archives of Physical Medicine and Rehabilitation 64: 237–242
Robertson E S 1971 How independent is the limb deficient child? Occupational Therapy Today–Tomorrow. Proceedings of the 5th International Congress of the World Federation of Occupational Therapy, Zurich, p 107–112
Sauter W F 1991 The use of electric elbows in the rehabilitation of children with upper limb deficiencies. Prosthetics and Orthotics International 15: 93–95
Sorbye E 1977 Myoelectric controlled hand prostheses in children. International Journal of Rehabilitation Research 1: 15–25
Trial of the Swedish Myoelectric Hand for young children. 1981 DHSS, London, Summarized in Physiotherapy 67(10): 312
Trost F J 1983 A comparison of conventional and myoelectric below-elbow prosthetic use. Inter Clinic Information Bulletin 18(4): 9–16
Van Lunteren A, Van Lunteren-Gerritsen G H M, Stassen H G, Zuithoff M J 1983 A field evaluation of arm prostheses for unilateral amputees. Prosthetics and Orthotics International 7: 141–151

18. General advice to the amputee

The following advice is given to new amputees before discharge and is applicable throughout their whole life.

CARE OF THE STUMP

Hygiene

The amputee is made aware that there may be increased perspiration over the whole area of the stump that is encased in the prosthesis. Skin problems may occur if meticulous stump hygiene is not carried out.

The stump should be washed daily with soap and water, preferably in the evening. A damp stump pushed into a socket in the morning can cause skin damage. The stump must be dried thoroughly, with particular attention being paid to skin folds. Oil, cream or spirit should not be applied to the skin. In hot weather the stump will need to be washed and dried several times a day.

The skin of the stump must be examined daily, using a mirror where necessary. If there is a problem with the skin of the stump, the following points must be considered:

— *The stump sock*: This must be clean and correctly pulled up so that there are no wrinkles inside the socket. Some amputees may have a skin sensitivity to wool or nylon.
— *The prosthesis*: A correct fit is essential.
— *The skin*: If there is a distinct skin problem, the amputee must seek medical advice; simple remedies are often successful but occasionally advice must be sought from a consultant dermatologist. This is needed, in particular, for allergic and fungal skin conditions.

Stump complications

Examples are as follows:

— Open areas
— Sinuses
— Bone infections
— Exostoses
— Dermatitis
— Oedema with suspected underlying pathology
— Soft tissue lesions
— Necrosis
— Neuroma.

Often complications occur as a result of an ill-fitting prosthesis. The physiotherapist can carry out simple measures to correct them, but it may be necessary for the doctor and prosthetist in the DSC to carry out major adjustments or order a new prosthesis. Both the physiotherapist and the amputee must be aware that seemingly minor stump problems can escalate drastically if they are not dealt with promptly. Occasionally it may be necessary to refer amputees back to their hospital surgeon.

CARE OF THE REMAINING LIMB

All amputees need to be aware that their ability to walk depends on the condition of the remaining limb. This is particularly vital for those suffering from peripheral vascular disease (PVD) and diabetes.

Hygiene

The foot and leg should be washed daily with warm water and mild soap. After rinsing thoroughly, careful drying must be carried out and a soft towel used to blot in between the toes. The skin should not be vigorously rubbed. The district nurse or carer should be asked to carry out this procedure if the patient is unable to do so.

Toe nails should be cut with great care. After bathing, the nail is softer and easier to manage. The edge should be cut following the shape of the toe; the corners of the nails should never be cut back into the nail grooves. The nails should not be cut too short. If there is any difficulty a qualified chiropodist must be consulted.

When the amputee is sitting down for a short rest at home it is advisable to elevate the leg on a stool; this prevents oedema. The legs must not be crossed. The heel should be protected with a sheepskin heel cushion to avoid heel ulceration from concentrated pressure.

Peripheral neuropathy

One of the main problems for the diabetic patient is peripheral neuropathy. No opportunity should be lost by physiotherapists, nurses or chiropodists to emphasise the danger of this lack of sensation to the patient.

The following advice must be given:

— Visually check the remaining foot daily. If the amputee has visual impairment the check should be made by a relative or district nurse.
— Use a thermometer to test the temperature of bath water, which must not exceed 40°C.
— Avoid hot water bottles; wrap a warm rug around the leg in bed. Similarly, do not sit close to a fire; use a rug instead.
— Avoid sunburn to the lower leg.
— Check the inside of shoes daily for foreign bodies or protruding tacks, nails, etc.
— Never wear new shoes for longer than 2 hours to begin with, even if they have been made to measure.
— Do not try instant foot 'cures' advertised in newspapers as they rarely work.
— If the foot gets wet, it must be dried thoroughly and put into dry hose and shoes.
— Corn pads, plasters and other dressings should not be applied without the advice of a chiropodist.

Chiropody

The chiropodist will diagnose foot disorders, implement treatment programmes, relieve foot pain and provide advice on footwear and footcare.

The amputee must only seek the advice of a state registered chiropodist (SRCh), who may work within the NHS or be in private practice. Those suffering from diabetes, PVD and rheumatoid arthritis must be seen regularly by a chiropodist. The elderly who cannot attend to their own foot care must also have their feet checked regularly, either by the chiropodist or district nurse.

Chiropody services are provided free of charge to the following priority groups:

— Expectant and nursing mothers
— Diabetics not of pensionable age
— Children, 0–18 years
— Men of pensionable age
— Women of pensionable age
— Physically handicapped
— Mentally handicapped
— Medical need, e.g. rheumatoid arthritis, registered blind, etc; patients in this category require referral from the GP or consultant.

Most large hospitals have a chiropodist who will treat patients considered to be at risk and who have been referred by a consultant; these patients include diabetics and those with PVD, etc. In the community, chiropody treatment is usually carried out in health centres and there is a domiciliary service for the housebound. The patient's GP can generally supply details about local facilities. Conditions commonly dealt with by the chiropodist include:

— Corns
— Bunions
— Callosities
— Ingrowing toenails
— Thick horny toenails
— Skin problems on the foot
— Toe and foot deformities.

The chiropodist must contact the amputee's GP or hospital doctor if there are any untoward signs in the remaining foot. There are various leaflets available from the Society of Chiropodists (53 Welbeck Street, London W1M 7HE) on the care of the foot.

Footwear

Socks or stockings should not be pulled tightly over the toes, and should not have a restrictive elasticated top or be supported by a garter or elastic band. They must be washed daily. Natural fibres are preferable to nylon.

Shoes must be well fitting, in a good state of repair and not too rigid. A natural material such as leather or canvas is advisable as it permits the foot to 'breathe'. Strappy sandals should be avoided as these cause lesions when the foot swells, particularly in the summer. There are many shoes available, either from shops or hospital appliance departments, which have a wide range of widths, depths and weight to suit individual needs. It may take a great deal of effort from the amputee, physiotherapist, occupational therapist or chiropodist to find suitably comfortable and cosmetically acceptable footwear. This must be pursued with great vigour to achieve good results.

If the amputee or physiotherapist observes any untoward signs or symptoms in the remaining foot or leg, a doctor must be consulted immediately.

Backcare

Footwear and heel height can alter the alignment of the prosthesis, which in turn may affect the lumbar spine, particularly in the transfemoral levels and above. Shoes must be kept in a good state of repair; badly worn soles and heels cause a change in the alignment. The height of the heel of the shoe should not be changed from that for which the prosthesis was designed, unless the prosthesis has an adjustable foot (see Ch. 7), as this also alters the alignment. If an amputee presents with back pain, both musculoskeletal and prosthetic causes should be investigated.

Strength and mobility

The amputee must be taught a regime of maintenance exercises for the hip, knee and foot of the remaining limb. The elderly should perform these exercises daily. Other amputees need to re-start this exercise programme if they are forced to rest for a period of time because of illness or fitting problems with the prosthesis. The community physiotherapist may need to visit these patients at home, or the amputee may need to re-attend the physiotherapy department (see Ch. 4).

CARE OF THE PROSTHESIS

Whenever the amputee has any queries concerning the fit, length, suspension, mechanical function or general state of repair of the prosthesis, the prosthetist must be contacted. Alterations or repairs should not be carried out by the amputee. The amputee is never discharged from the care of the prosthetic service.

If either the foot or knee mechanism becomes wet or clogged with dust or foreign material, the limb must be checked. The patient should not walk in water without special protective covering. Swimming must not be attempted in an ordinary prosthesis.

If the amputee has a fall, particularly one which involves the prosthesis, this should be checked immediately by the prosthetist for safety, even if there appears to be no damage.

The prosthetic foot must be regularly checked for wear with the shoe and sock removed, particularly in the case of heavy and active users.

Cleaning

Any metal or plastic socket should be wiped clean with a damp cloth at night and then dried. Soap should not be used.

Leather sockets cannot be cleaned; they may need to be renewed frequently. The thigh corset, in particular, needs renewing if the patient is incontinent or sweats excessively.

The liners of PTB and PTS prostheses can be wiped with a damp cloth but they may need frequent renewal. Liners made of PELite can be washed with soap flakes, rinsed out and hung up to dry away from direct heat.

The valve of the suction socket (see Ch. 11) must be kept free from dust with a small soft brush, as powder and dust can collect in it. Cross-threading must be avoided.

Body weight

Any change in the amputee's body weight will cause an alteration in the fit of the socket. This can be a particular problem when weight increase produces a tight socket.

The obese patient finds it more difficult to use a prosthesis skillfully and effectively, e.g. bulging fatty tissue in the adductor region causes discomfort and chafing.

Those who lose weight will find that the socket becomes far too loose and requires adjustment. The method of suspension may need to be altered. All bony prominences should be checked for rubbing.

CARE OF THE STUMP SOCK

A clean, dry stump sock should be worn daily. During hot weather stump socks may need to be changed more than once a day. Some very active limb users may need to do this in cooler weather as well.

The socks should be washed by hand. Soap flakes should be used, never biological detergents. Lukewarm water should be used and thorough rinsing is necessary to remove all of the soap. The socks should be dried flat on a towel, away from direct heat. Spin dryers and tumble dryers shrink the socks and mat the fibres.

The amputee must be aware of the several types of stump sock available; sometimes different combinations of materials need to be tried out to achieve a comfortable fit (see Ch. 7).

INFORMATION

Local DSCs supply a wide range of information leaflets and can provide advice on all aspects of aftercare for the amputee.

REFERENCES

Barnett A, Odugbesan O 1987 Foot care for diabetics. Nursing Times 83 (22): 24–26

Brooks A P 1981 The diabetic foot. Hospital Update May: 509–514

Disabled Living Foundation 1991 Footwear: a quality issue. Disabled Living Foundation, London

Finlay O E 1986 Footwear management in the elderly care programme. Physiotherapy 72 (4): 172–178

Hoile R 1981 Managing the ischaemic limb in the community. Community View 10: 10–12

Levy S W 1980 Skin problems of the leg amputee. Prosthetics and Orthotics International 4 (1): 37–44

Stokes I A F 1977 The effect of shoe inserts on the load distribution under the foot. Chiropodist January: 5–12

19. The problem of pain

Pain is a complex physiological phenomenon which is unusually difficult to define in precise terms, but it has some clearly discernible characteristics. It is an unpleasant sensory and emotional experience commanding a response, which, even when not expressed verbally, may be reflected in the individual's behaviour and often in other physical signs.

In this chapter the authors do not attempt to describe the neurophysiological basis of pain and its perception; these can be fully read elsewhere (see References and Bibliography). However, included here is practical information related to the everyday care of the amputee. The reason for pain may be physical (resulting from tissue disturbance or damage), psychological, or an intricate combination of both. The pain may be acute, chronic, intermittent, constant or triggered by a specific action.

The amputee may report that pain is felt in the stump, or may localise it to the 'phantom limb'. The amputee may feel pain in a phantom limb with normal anatomy, or the foot may be located abnormally, i.e. proximally or in a strange position, such as twisted. Pain in the phantom limb is not an imaginary phenomenon, even though it is felt in parts of a limb that are not present.

It should be recognised that the assessment of pain is best made with a multidisciplinary team, i.e. therapists, nurses, doctor, clinical psychologists, etc. The underlying causes of any pain must be recognised, investigated thoroughly and explained so that appropriate treatment is instituted by the team member best able to do this. It should be remembered that pain control should be achieved prior to surgery, when the patient is having pre-operative investigations.

For the amputee, pain may be present early after the operation, and occasionally becomes a longstanding problem when it remains. This same pain can recur or a new pain may present months or even years after a pain-free post-amputation period.

EARLY DISCOMFORT

Adverse reactions of the patient to postoperative pain can be minimised by effective pre- and postoperative analgesia. In addition, the ability of patients to talk freely about their feelings regarding the surgery to a team member with an understanding ear and an ability to answer questions will diminish the fear of pain. However, all patients experience discomfort in the early postoperative period and this may be caused by the following:

1. In the immediate postoperative phase, discomfort or pain is felt in the wound site and oedematous tissues. Excessive early pain may be caused by a haematoma; increasing pain 2–3 days after surgery may result from a developing infection.

2. Occasionally, the active exercise programme in the physiotherapy department may cause discomfort in muscles and joints unaccustomed to movement and stretching.

3. During prosthetic rehabilitation, both when the early walking aid is used and during the initial weeks of using the first prosthesis, the stump may become sore from the new pressures exerted on the tissues.

4. All amputees have an awareness of the phantom of a limb postoperatively. This phantom

sensation is felt following the loss of any non-visceral part of the body, e.g. mastectomy, as well as after amputation of a limb. This is due to the persistence of nerve impulses travelling through the nerve fibres and synapses relating to the amputated part, and to the memory of such a part in the higher levels of the central nervous system.

Phantom sensation may be experienced to a greater degree soon after the amputation, but will tend to fade gradually with time, as memory fades and the impulses adapt to the new situation. Sensory re-education must be started from the first postoperative day (see Ch. 3), with the patient becoming accustomed to light pressure first and, as time progresses, to handling and resisted exercise.

If the patient complains of phantom pain during this early period it should be treated immediately to prevent it from becoming a chronic problem.

All these types of discomfort are understandable and very common. The physiotherapist, through a positive approach to rehabilitation with reassurance and explanation to the patient, can be invaluable in alleviating anxiety.

Simple remedies for these discomforts include:

— Explanation that most of these early problems are temporary
— Careful graduation of the rehabilitation programme in respect of pain
— Request for an alteration of the fit or alignment of the prosthesis
— Re-evaluation of the amputee's daily management
— Re-adjustment of analgesia
— Diversionary recreational activities.

LATER PAIN PROBLEMS

Generally speaking, the majority of patients will have adapted to life as an amputee by the time they have become mobile with their first prosthesis. This means that they will have learned to cope with the early discomforts and adjustments and will have started to discover their potential. However, there are a few patients who still complain repeatedly of either stump or phantom pain: this will have been a problem from the start, despite the trial of simple remedies as described above. Also, there is a group of patients who have initially experienced no problems of this sort, but who present at a later stage complaining of pain.

Causes of later pain problems

Physical

— Scar contracture
— Unhealed wound
— Oedema
— Neuroma
— Bony spur
— Pain referred, e.g. from the lumbar spine or abdominal viscera
— Ischaemic or claudication pain of the amputated side
— Arthritic conditions
— Neurological abnormalities, e.g. hemiplegia, spina bifida, diabetes mellitus
— Fracture
— Regrowth of tumour
— Adverse neural tension.

Psychological

— *Anxiety*: this, accompanied by depression, will make physical pain harder to bear.
— *Hysteria*: wishing to maintain the 'patient' status may appear to some individuals a way of gaining attention; there may possibly be other underlying causes.
— *Poor adjustment*: patients who, even prior to amputation, have adjusted poorly to their social, occupational or marital lives are unlikely to perform better after it and may use this as an excuse.
— *Non-adjustment*: the whole experience and history of the events leading up to and following the amputation can influence the patient's adjustment to the discomfort of being an amputee.
— *Culture*: cultural influences of different races play some part in the experience of pain.
— *Compensation cases*: the influence of possible litigation in the matter concerning the cause

and outcome of amputation can affect certain individuals.

— *Lack of medical sympathy*: some individuals may persist in their complaints of pain if they consider they are being ignored.

Very often strong pain can result from a continuation of both physical and psychological factors and it can be dangerous to classify a patient as having a 'psychological problem' without meticulous physical assessment. In some cases where there is litigation pending, it may be difficult to treat the patient's pain successfully until the legal proceedings have been completed.

MANAGEMENT OF PAIN

A multidisciplinary approach, a sympathetic attitude and an intelligent understanding of the causes of pain, as well as the use of the various methods of treatment available, will in most cases help patients overcome the unpleasant experience of their pain.

Physiotherapy

The physiotherapist is frequently one of the first team members approached with the problem and must consider every aspect of pain while assessing the amputee. This assessment may be carried out with the use of pain charts, pain questionnaires, a diary in which patients can record their own pain pattern, or by careful questioning.

It must be realised that assessment in these cases cannot take place in one out-patient session but that it may take a number of sessions to investigate a possible cause for the pain or to formulate an accurate impression of the problem. Only by observation of the patient over a period of time will an accurate picture emerge. At some hospitals, the assessment is carried out by out-patient visits and, at others, the patient is admitted for a period of time.

Subjective examination

The nature of the pain must be known and recorded. Is it, for instance, nagging, burning, dull, sharp, intermittent or constant? At what time of day is the pain felt? What aggravates or relieves the pain? Where is the exact site of pain? Is it originating from the phantom limb, or stump, or both? Is there any radiation? Is there any paraesthesia? Is the patient's sleep disturbed by pain?

What is the lifestyle of the amputee? The type of medication and the frequency with which it is taken, the amount of tobacco and alcohol consumed, the type of social interaction amputees have and whether they are able to work, are all relevant pieces of information.

Objective examination

1. Observation and palpation is undertaken of:

— The tissues of the stump
— The pulses in the affected leg
— All the joints of the affected limb (and test of its muscle strength)
— The cervical, thoracic, lumbar spine, as pain can be referred distally.

2. The fit and alignment of the prosthesis during all activities is examined.
3. The general state of hygiene and physical fitness of the patient is assessed.

The possible underlying cause of the amputee's pain can be assessed by the physiotherapist, both from this formal assessment and from an informal observation of the patient during activities of daily living over a period of time. A medical opinion should then be sought for a diagnosis to be made following further investigation. Sometimes, it may take weeks or months for a diagnosis to be confirmed, and only after a period of trial and error with various treatments.

Treatment by the physiotherapist

The physiotherapist should undertake treatment for stump or phantom pain where there is evidence of physical mechanisms occurring which may be influenced by physical treatments. In certain circumstances, it may also be necessary to use physiotherapy in combination with psychological or psychiatric treatments, if the whole team, after careful evaluation, considers it to be appropriate. It is also the physiotherapist's responsibility to check the fit of the prosthesis, its state of repair and the type of socks used, and refer the patient back to the DSC if the pain experienced relates to a problem with the prosthesis.

There are many treatment modalities which can be effective, but whichever is selected must be given a reasonable trial before stopping, modifying or changing to another modality. Clear records must be kept of each treatment used, the individual technique employed and the patient's response.

The following treatments are merely suggestions: individual techniques and preferences vary. The accepted contra-indications for these modalities apply to the amputee as for all patients.

Oedema control techniques and tissue support

Where the stump pain is seen to be caused by oedema, a variety of methods of treatment are available (see Ch. 3). Occasionally, merely a sensation of contained tissue support is required. A bandage can be used or a 'night socket'. This can be made of Plastazote in the physiotherapy department, or made by the prosthetist using other materials.

Transcutaneous nerve stimulation

As the optimal positioning of the electrodes, frequency of current and duration of treatment can take some time to determine, the patient must be prepared to attend daily as an outpatient or be admitted to hospital. Charts should be kept to record pain site and severity, electrode placement and frequency of use, time and duration of treatment and the effect produced. If this treatment shows signs of success, the patient can be supplied with a machine for home use, but only if a regular re-assessment follow-up programme is in operation.

Ultrasound

This can be given if there is reason to believe that soft tissue structures are the cause of pain. If some improvement has not been achieved within four treatments it is unlikely to succeed.

Thermal modalities

Ice packs, heat (in a variety of forms) or contrast techniques can be used.

Percussion

A small rubber hammer, an electrical vibrator or manual techniques can be used. Percussion is best employed while the patient is experiencing pain; it should not be used during the periods of freedom from pain.

Spinal treatment

Where there is stump pain which is reproducible on spinal movements, treatments such as mobilisation or manipulation, traction, exercise, etc. are appropriate.

Peripheral joints

Where joint range limitations exist, appropriate mobilising modalities should be carried out. Adverse neural tension can be relieved by mobilising the neural tissue.

Other treatments

Acupuncture, electro-acupuncture, megapulse, laser and interferential therapy have also been reported as giving some relief for stump pain, but the authors have no experience of this.

Medical treatment

Pharmacological

— Non-opiate analgesia
— Anti-inflammatory agents
— Vasodilators
— Muscle relaxants
— Antidepressants
— Injections: these may be in the form of a sensory nerve block, a sympathetic block or anti-inflammatory injections.

Surgical

— Excision of neuroma
— Revision of scar

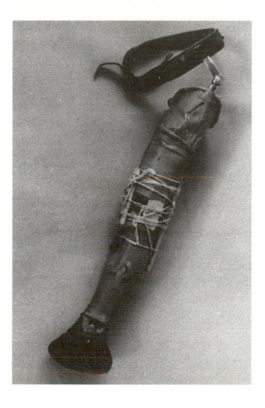 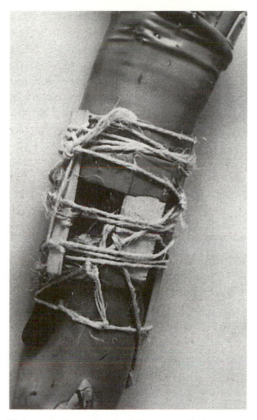

Fig. 19.1 One patient's attempted cure for phantom pain. This particular patient had phantom pain but was convinced that there were 'little devils' in the artificial limb causing the trouble. He attacked these by beating the limb and sticking nails into it. He then had to 'splint' the knee so that he was still able to walk.

— Trim of stump
— Trim of exostosis.

Psychological treatment

A skilled doctor, nurse, or medical social worker can often evaluate if there is a psychological problem at the root of the patient's complaint of pain, or acting as a compounding factor, and regular counselling over a period of time can sometimes help (see Ch. 2). There should be an overlap between the roles of the psychiatrist, psychologist, social worker, nurse and physiotherapist.

Clinical Psychologist

This profession will look into the behavioural pattern of the pain: what precipitates this pain; what are the consequences of it on the amputee's lifestyle and work; can it be altered? Evaluation, counselling, group therapy and hypnotherapy are techniques which may be employed.

An example of a problem that the clinical psychologist would deal with, would be a patient with a history of prolonged pain before amputation which has led to early phantom pain. The amputee's whole life setting must be explored with the psychologist and the indications are that rehabilitation may be prolonged and complicated.

Psychiatrist

This profession will deal with the patient with a serious depressive syndrome. This can manifest itself in loss of enjoyment of life, loss of sleep, loss of weight and change in mood. Frequently, patients who have made a good adjustment to their amputation but subsequently present years later complaining of pain, are those with a depressive illness. The pain experienced may be part of this depressive syndrome, or a depression may become much worse if there is severe physical pain present. This syndrome is treated by drug therapy. Very often these patients will respond better if the drug treatment is combined with other physical treatments.

CONCLUSION

The management of pain is not easy. It will require precise evaluation by many different professions and intricate combinations of treatment over a period of time. However, it is advisable that one team member has overall responsibility for a patient so that continuity is maintained.

It must be remembered that, whatever the cause, this pain is real to the patient and can totally disrupt both the amputee's life and that of family and friends. However, both stump and phantom pain tend to be cyclic in nature, with spontaneous remission and relapses.

A few stump and phantom pains cannot be relieved. These are very difficult for patients and for those looking after them. An effort must then be made to get the patient to accept the pain as part of life and to continue living as normally as possible in spite of it. No patient should be labelled 'psychological' and dismissed without help or support, whatever the real cause may be. Whichever drug or treatment method helps most should be used and the patient should not 'shop around' hospital after hospital for a 'magic' cure (see Fig. 19.1).

REFERENCES

Berger S M 1980 Conservative management of phantom limb and amputation-stump pain. Annals of the Royal College of Surgeons 62: 103–105

Connolly J 1979 Phantom and stump pain following operation. Physiotherapy 65(1): 13–14

Doliber C M 1984 Role of the physical therapist at pain treatment centres. Physical Therapy 64(6): 905–909

Feldman R S 1983 Phantom limb pain. Blesmag Spring: 19–21

Frampton V M 1982 Pain control with the aid of transcutaneous nerve stimulation. Physiotherapy 68(3): 77–81

Hittenberger D A 1982 Use of electric stimulation in prosthetics for the control of pain. Orthotics and Prosthetics 36(2): 35–41

Kristen H, Lukeschitsch G, Plattner F, Sigmund R, Resch P 1984 Thermography as a means for quantitative assessment of stump and phantom pains. Prosthetics and Orthotics International 8(2): 76–81

Lewith George T 1981 Acupuncture. World of Medicine Update 509–520

Melzack R 1975 The McGill pain questionnaire: major properties and scoring methods. Pain 1: 277–299

Melzack R, Wall P D 1965 Pain mechanisms: a new theory. Science 150(3699): 971–979

Monga T N, Jaksic T 1981 Acupuncture in phantom limb pain. Archives of Physical Medicine and Rehabilitation 62: 229–231

Mouratoglou V M 1986 Amputees and phantom limb pain: a literature review. Physiotherapy Practice 2(4): 177–185

Ottoson D, Lundeberg S 1985 Conservative management of painful stumps in the upper limb amputee. Newsletter of the British Association of Hand Therapists (January)

Parkes C M 1973 Factors determining the persistence of phantom pain in the amputee. Journal of Psychosomatic Research 17: 97–108

Reading A E 1980 A comparison of pain rating scales. Journal of Psychosomatic Research 24: 119–124

Sacks O 1986 Phantoms. In: The man who mistook his wife for a hat. Picador, London, Ch 6

Sedgwick E M 1991 Phantom limbs. Step Forward Issue 25 (winter)

Steinbach T V, Nadvorna H, Arazi D 1982 A five year follow-up study of phantom limb pain in post traumatic amputees. Scandinavian Journal of Rehabilitation Medicine 14: 203–207

Swerdlow M 1980 The treatment of shooting pain. Postgraduate Medical Journal 56: 159–161

Wall P D 1980 The gate control theory of pain mechanisms — a re-examination and restatement. Brain 101: 1–18

Wall P D, Devor S 1981 The effect of peripheral nerve injury on dorsal root potentials and on transmission of afferent signals into the spinal cord. Brain Research 209: 95–111

Withrington R H, Wynn Parry C B 1984 The management of painful peripheral nerve disorders. Journal of Hand Surgery 9B(1): 24–28

Wyke B D 1981 Neurological aspects of pain therapy: a review of some current concepts. In: Swerdlow M (ed) The therapy of pain. MTP Press, Lancaster

Wynn Parry C B 1981 The 1981 Philip Nichols Memorial Lecture. International Rehabilitation Medicine 4: 59–65

Wynn Parry C B 1984 The management of painful peripheral nerve disorders. In: Wall P D, Melzack R (eds) Textbook of pain. Churchill Livingstone, Edinburgh, p 395–401

20. Special cases

Patients who have undergone an amputation may well have other medical problems. These medical problems may be apparent before the amputation, or may appear years afterwards. In the case of those suffering from peripheral vascular disease and diabetes, there are obvious associated problems which have already been discussed (see Chs 2 and 3).

Younger amputees may experience other medical problems as they grow older, or, if the amputation was caused by severe trauma, they may have other injuries associated with that trauma. Additional complications may be caused by these medical problems or injuries when patients are wearing prostheses, and the physiotherapist should be aware of the difficulties which may occur. There are no rigid rules concerning these types of patients, and each will have to be considered, assessed and treated individually.

Some of these special cases are described in this chapter.

HEMIPLEGIA

Amputation with hemiplegia is a common combination of problems. Mobility will depend on the severity and time of onset of the stroke, the level of amputation and (most importantly) whether the stroke and amputation affect opposite sides. Careful evaluation at the pre-operative stage and postoperatively with the Ppam aid or Femurett will help in the assessment of whether prosthetic rehabilitation is indicated. Positive rehabilitation in a wheelchair must be given whether the amputee is supplied with a prosthesis or not, and the home situation should be re-assessed.

The stroke and the amputation on the same side

Successful prosthetic rehabilitation may be possible if the amputation is at an above-knee level. Below-knee amputations are unsuccessful prosthetically because of insufficient muscle control at the knee joint and altered tone. The through-knee amputee with marked increase in flexor tone at the hip has similar problems, as flexion cannot be accommodated in the long socket (see Ch. 12).

The stroke and the amputation on opposite sides

Prosthetic rehabilitation is sometimes successful with the lower levels of amputation, i.e. Symes or below-knee, but this applies only if there is an uncomplicated postoperative course and a prosthesis is supplied as soon as possible.

Bilateral amputation followed by stroke

Hemiplegic amputees require a simple lightweight prosthesis with easy fastenings using Velcro attachments. Prosthetic re-education should not cause too many difficulties; walking aids are chosen according to their suitability for each patient. Learning to apply and remove the prosthesis may be a problem for the patient, and it may be necessary for a carer to learn the procedures in order to be able to help.

If these patients have amputations above the knee joint on the stroke side and have been competent prosthetic users before the stroke, it is possible for them to continue using prostheses. This is because the prosthetic knee joint can lock and provide stability on the weaker side. However, overall management should be very carefully considered and the energy cost of mobility taken into account. Wheelchair independence and home assessments must be completed before prostheses are considered.

The established amputee suffering a stroke

Amputation and a stroke may occur within a short space of time, particularly in those patients suffering from arterial disease. However, there is a small number of longstanding amputees who experience strokes during their latter years. The same rules for the success of prosthetic rehabilitation regarding side of amputation and side of stroke apply here as just described, although these amputees usually walk extremely well after recovery from the initial neurological disturbance. Sometimes the prosthesis may require alteration, especially in the case of the above-knee amputee walking with a free knee gait pattern.

SPINA BIFIDA

Teenagers or young adults who are able to walk with boots and calipers may find that, as they mature, their hyposensitive feet, or chronic ulceration, are unacceptable. The orthoses may be heavy and appear urgainly. Below-knee amputation may be considered in these cases, to increase mobility and improve cosmesis. However, it is essential that this decision is taken only after careful consideration by both the orthopaedic surgeon and the rehabilitation consultant, and after the patient has had the opportunity to visit the DSC to look at prostheses (see combined clinic, Ch. 1).

Careful assessment and recording of the patient's muscle power and skin sensation is important to evaluate whether knee function will be adequate to use a prosthesis.

Spina bifida patients need careful gait rehabilitation and this should be carried out where there is immediate prosthetic help. In many cases, although muscle power is reasonable there may be unequal muscle pull, which creates some torsion and friction at the stump/socket interface. As skin sensation may be imperfect, the physio-

therapist must check the skin constantly and teach the patient to carry out the same procedure. If there are any rubs or soreness, the socket must be adjusted immediately by the prosthetist and the skin must return to normal before gait re-education recommences.

Walking aids will again be chosen for each individual. Usually there is little problem in using the prostheses, as these patients are already familiar with orthoses and are extremely capable.

Hygiene and care of the stump and prosthesis should be explained in detail (see Ch. 18) as many of these patients have problems with sweating and incontinence.

PARAPLEGIA

Occasionally a paraplegic patient may require an amputation. Gross ischaemia, fractures which are impossible to stabilise and extensive infection may be life endangering, and after many months of treatment amputation of the affected part may be the only treatment left.

These patients rarely use prostheses. It is sometimes difficult for the patient to appreciate this, particularly if long leg calipers had been used before the amputation. Both the doctor and the physiotherapist must explain to the patient that skin tolerance and pressure sensitivity is vital for the use of any prosthesis. It may be necessary to retrain sitting balance, transfers and general wheelchair independence.

BURNED SKIN/GRAFTED SKIN

The skin of amputees with burns or grafts must be carefully examined when they are using prostheses. Any tissue abnormality which produces poor sensation, adhesions, lack of viability or frank breakdown is potentially dangerous for those using prostheses. The patient must be aware of this problem and know how to check pressure areas of the socket.

Care is needed with the timing of the first trial of the early walking aid and the fitting of the prosthesis, so that skin tolerance to pressure is gradually built up. If minor skin breakdown occurs initially, it is advisable to wait a little longer, possibly 2 weeks, before carrying out another trial.

Frequently the first prosthesis may be very basic. Progression to more sophisticated prostheses is possible if the skin toughens adequately, but this can often take more than 1 year. These patients must not become disheartened and may require frequent attendances at their local DSC for psychological support and prosthetic adjustment.

THE BLIND AND PARTIALLY SIGHTED

Diabetes mellitus is a common cause of visual handicap amongst amputees. Successful prosthetic rehabilitation will depend on whether the blindness is long-standing and whether the patient's mobility is already well adjusted to it. These patients are usually extremely capable of coping with their situation and, once the prosthesis is understood, gait rehabilitation must be aimed at full weight-bearing. This is because the patient will need a hand free to use a white stick to locate obstacles or to hold a guide-dog's harness. Two walking sticks would therefore be impractical and cumbersome.

The less fortunate blind amputees are those whose sight is gradually diminishing at the same time as the amputation occurs. Both situations are extremely difficult for the patient to cope with and progress is slow.

The fit and the feel of the prosthesis must be carefully explained and the physiotherapist must initially check the weightbearing areas constantly. Later, it may be necessary to explain this procedure to carers and teach them how to observe and check the fit of the prosthesis, particularly if there is hyposensitivity in the stump. Simple fastenings will be required. Once a correct fit of the prosthesis has been achieved and initial mobility mastered in the physiotherapy department, it is more relevant for gait re-education to continue in the home, with the community physiotherapist supervising the treatment programme.

THE DEAF AND THOSE WITH VESTIBULAR DISORDERS

Balance problems should be assessed prior to prosthetic use and intensive rehabilitation should be given.

Carers of the profoundly deaf may have to be called on to attend the physiotherapy department during prosthetic rehabilitation if communication with the patient is difficult.

The hard of hearing occasionally have flat batteries in their hearing aids and it is useful to have some spares in the physiotherapy department. Some patients may benefit from an assessment in the ear, nose and throat department of the hospital as minor problems, such as excessive wax, can be quickly dealt with.

COLOSTOMY

When a patient with a colostomy needs an amputation, it is important that particular attention is given to the design of the suspension of the prosthesis prior to prescription. It may be necessary that the position of waist or pelvic suspension is adjusted to accommodate the colostomy. Similar consideration should be given to the types of suspension required for patients with hernias, particularly for those wearing a support.

Patients suffering from gross trauma requiring an amputation and a colostomy are often able to use prostheses. At Roehampton there have been several patients with hip disarticulation and a colostomy who have managed well. Expert help is required from the prosthetist during prosthetic re-education. It is advisable that these patients attend for physiotherapy in a unit where prosthetic services are available.

Occasionally an established amputee will need a colostomy. It is advisable that the surgeon observes the patient wearing the prosthesis and notes the position of the suspension used pre-operatively. The stoma created can then be placed clear of straps and belts; this makes the colostomy bag easier to manage. Alternatively, the surgeon can contact the rehabilitation consultant in order to discuss alteration of the suspension of the pros-thesis. The local stoma therapist may also need to give added support and advice to the amputee after discharge from hospital.

ARTHRODESED LOWER LIMB JOINTS

Arthrodesed lower limb joints can cause problems for the amputee during gait training. The mechanics of walking with a stiff knee or hip joint, either on the remaining leg or on the amputated leg with a prosthesis, can be extremely complicated, tiring and uncomfortable.

There are certain points to consider when assessing these patients pre-operatively. If the hip joint is arthrodesed on the side of the proposed amputation, the amount of flexion in the hip should be noted. It is not easy for an amputee to sit down or stand up wearing a prosthesis if the hip joint is fixed. The physiotherapist must check that the patient will have sufficient trunk flexion to reach down to the stump to apply the prosthesis, or that a carer is available to do this. If the knee joint is arthrodesed on the side of the proposed amputation, there is no benefit in carrying out a below-knee amputation.

When an amputee with an arthrodesed joint learns to walk with a prosthesis, standing up and sitting down must be checked. It may not be easy for an amputee with two stiff knee joints to sit in a normal chair, and chair, toilet and bed heights will require modification.

FRACTURES AND JOINT REPLACEMENTS

Those amputees with fractures in the lower limb generally have to wait until full weightbearing is permitted before they can use a prosthesis. It is therefore essential that an exercise programme is performed daily to strengthen muscles and preserve joint mobility. If the fracture is on the amputated side the stump will become oedematous; this oedema must have subsided considerably before a prosthetic fitting (see Ch. 3).

If the orthopaedic surgeon permits, the early walking aid can be used at the partial weight-bearing stage (see Ch. 5). Amputees must not attempt to remobilise in their existing prosthesis after a fracture, before the alignment and fit have been checked by the prosthetist, or a different prosthesis has been supplied with more proximal weightbearing areas.

Patients with hip arthroplasties are limited in their range of movement. The type of artificial limb supplied and the method of application will have to be carefully considered to avoid dislocation of the joint prosthesis.

PROGRESSIVE NEUROLOGICAL CONDITIONS

Amputees with neurological conditions such as multiple sclerosis, Parkinson's disease, motor neurone disease, etc., have complicated rehabilitation problems. During the early stages of these progressive conditions the physiotherapist may feel it is necessary to alter the type of walking aid. A frame may be more suitable if spasticity or balance problems are present, whereas Parkinson's disease sufferers may prefer to remain with walking sticks to maintain balance. All the problems that are associated with these conditions are more difficult because the patient also has to cope with a prosthesis. Obviously each case must be treated individually, but some may have to stop using the prosthesis because it becomes too difficult.

Wheelchair independence and functional capabilities in the activities of daily living should be re-assessed in the home. The physiotherapist, occupational therapist and social worker, both in the local hospital and community, must be aware of these patients and their problems in order that on-going help is available as new problems arise.

THE EXPERIENCED AMPUTEE ENCOUNTERING NEW PROBLEMS

This type of amputee is probably the most difficult case for the physiotherapist to manage. These amputees are expert prosthetic users, and know the prostheses and the system well. Unfortunately, as time progresses, the amputee, like everyone else, begins to encounter medical and physical problems that are associated with later life.

After a period of illness these amputees may find it difficult to use their prosthesis with exactly the same skill as before and become frustrated. This situation is often extremely difficult to explain and is not always accepted immediately. It may also be necessary to alter the prescription of the prosthesis. This calls for great tact and understanding on the part of the physiotherapist, prosthetist and all those caring for the patient.

CHILDREN AND ADOLESCENTS

The rehabilitation of children who have lower limb amputations will depend on their individual personality, age, developmental maturity and mood. Progress and gait pattern will depend upon age and maturity. When children are very small, provided that they can walk about with comfort, little attention need be given to the gait pattern. Frequent prosthetic appointments are needed to maintain the correct prescription. The parents must be aware of the fit and function of the prosthesis and should always attend the DSC with the child. As children mature, the gait pattern should improve and this pattern may change later, depending on the child's attitude.

It is not necessary to keep children attending for treatment on a regular basis, but each time the prescription of the prosthesis changes it is important to check that it is understood and used correctly. It may be necessary to visit the school and speak to teachers about realistic walking distances, sports and activities that the individual can undertake (see Ch. 15).

See also Chapter 2, congenital deformity.

DEPRESSION

Occasionally amputees, like anybody else, may suffer from depression; if this occurs it may be extremely difficult to treat. The depression may manifest itself in different ways. The prosthesis may be blamed, with the patient complaining of different aspects of its design, fit and comfort. Alternatively, the amputee appears unbalanced, walks with an extraordinary gait pattern and produces uncoordinated movements. Provided that the physiotherapist has checked the fit of the prosthesis and is happy with the amputee's physical capabilities, the patient should be referred for further help (see Ch. 19).

MULTIPLE AMPUTATIONS

Young people who have experienced gross trauma, or who are suffering from Buerger's disease, resulting in multiple loss of limbs, will need to attend a specialised centre with expert arm training facilities.

Those with bilateral lower limb amputations or a one upper/one lower limb combination, have the lower limb prostheses fitted first, and independence in walking is gained before arm training begins.

Those with bilateral upper limb amputations remain in a wheelchair and concentrate first on arm training with prostheses.

For multiple amputees, independence in the activities of daily living is of primary importance, and how this is achieved may or may not be with the assistance of prostheses. Careful assessment involving the rehabilitation consultant, the occupational therapist, the physiotherapist and the patient with his family is essential.

LEPROSY (HANSEN'S DISEASE)

Leprosy takes two principal forms: tuberculoid and lepromatous. Between these forms, the disease covers a broad spectrum.

In the tuberculoid form the skin shows areas of poor pigmentation bordered by roughened areas, and is anaesthetic. Patients are also likely to have nerve damage because the body's defence mechanism is so strong it destroys the nerve. In the lepromatous form the bacteria spreads everywhere and is responsible for the nerve destruction in regions such as the hands, feet and face. The skin is also affected with nodules resembling large blisters. It is a feature of leprosy bacteria that they grow in the cooler parts of the body, particularly exposed skin.

Leprosy was endemic in the UK until the eighteenth century; the last case died in 1798. Today, the disease is only contracted abroad; but 15–20 new cases present in the UK each year, one case requiring amputation every 4–5 years. In the developing world more amputations are performed as people walk a great deal, over longer distances and rough terrain, on anaesthetic feet often without protective footwear, thus causing greater damage.

At present, leprosy is treated with a combination of drugs which have revolutionised management of the disease. Patients are now able to be treated in general hospitals without segregation and, most importantly, the disease process can be stopped and so physical rehabilitation of deformities can be carried out.

These patients may require very distal amputations, e.g. one or two digits, and every effort should be made to achieve healing in cases of chronic ulceration of the anaesthetic foot before resorting to formal below-knee amputation.

However, if amputation is unavoidable because of bone destruction, long-term failure to heal, or risk of malignant change in the ulcer, these patients do run a very high risk of damage to the stump. The stump skin is often anaesthetic, especially in lepromatous patients, although some tuberculoids may have normal sensation if their anaesthetic skin lesion did not extend as far as the proximal part of the leg. In old lepromatous patients, in addition to anaesthesia, the stump skin quality may be very poor as a result of past lepromatous infiltration in the skin. Therefore, the skin of the stump may very easily be traumatised, both from pressure and from shearing strains, and it is important to test the stump for its areas of sensory loss. The prosthesis must therefore be very carefully fitted, and the stump and the prosthesis both require frequent checking. When the prosthesis is first supplied, and very carefully checked, the patient must be taught to use it carefully, initially by graded and limited walking.

Certainly in a Third World situation, patients will have great problems working and supporting their families if they cannot be fitted with prostheses. In addition, those patients who also have sensory loss over their hands, are likely to injure their hands should they attempt to use crutches long-term.

PROBLEMS ASSOCIATED WITH MENSTRUATION AND PREGNANCY

Some females suffer from a 'pre-menstrual syndrome', one facet of which is a feeling of fluid retention. In some amputees this can affect the size of the stump and the fit of the socket for a few days every month. This is more noticeable with the more intimately fitting sockets, such as the patellar tendon bearing socket and above-knee suction socket, and may be so severe as to prevent the patient from wearing these prostheses for those few days.

It is often the female physiotherapist who is first made aware of this problem as patients may find this difficult to discuss if they have a male doctor or prosthetist. Referral to a gynaecologist for systemic treatment may be required if simple methods of socket adjustment are unsuccessful. There is now more knowledge and understanding of the pre-menstrual syndrome and methods of treating it. Occasionally, symptomatic treatment such as diuretics may help. Patients who are diabetic should seek the help of their physician who will need to monitor any treatment given.

The pregnant amputee will generally be advised by the obstetrician to remain as mobile as possible for as long as it is comfortable. This may mean frequent visits to the DSC for alteration of suspension straps and fabrication of new sockets as size increases. It must be realised that the centre of gravity in the pregnant female alters after 20–24 weeks and even the non-amputee has balance problems. Therefore, balance may be even harder to maintain for amputees, when they are wearing prostheses or using crutches. When prosthetic wear is no longer possible, crutch hopping can continue without causing any damage to the patient or fetus. An excellent activity to maintain general fitness during pregnancy is swimming.

This chapter is a summary of the authors' experience of treatment of these varied conditions over the years. However, physiotherapists must always remember that each individual amputee is a special case.

REFERENCES

Altner P C, Rusin J J, DeBoer A 1980 Rehabilitation of blind patients with lower extremity amputations. Archives of Physical Medicine and Rehabilitation 61: 82–84

Bernd L, Blasius K, Lukoschek M, Lucke R 1991 The autologous stump plasty. Treatment for bony overgrowth in juvenile amputees. Journal of Bone and Joint Surgery 73B (2): 203–206

Bowker J H, Rills B M, Ledbetter C A, Hunter G A, Holliday P 1981 Fractures in lower limbs with prior amputation. Journal of Bone and Joint Surgery 63A (6): 915–920

Clark G S, Naso F, Ditunno J F 1980 Marked bone spur formation in a burn amputee patient. Archives of Physical Medicine and Rehabilitation 61: 189–192

Grundy D J, Silver J R 1983 Amputation for peripheral vascular disease in the paraplegic and tetraplegic. Paraplegia 21: 305–311

Grundy D J, Silver J R 1984 Major amputation in paraplegic

and tetraplegic patients. International Rehabilitation Medicine 6: 162–165

LaBorde T C, Meier R H 1978 Amputations resulting from electrical injury: a review of 22 cases. Archives of Physical Medicine and Rehabilitation 59: 134–137

Malin A S et al 1991 Leprosy in reaction: a medical emergency. British Medical Journal 302: 1324–1326

Milling A W F 1984 Multiple traumatic limb amputations. Injury 16 (6): 6

Pfeil J et al 1991 The stump capping procedure to prevent or treat terminal osseous overgrowth. Prosthetics and Orthotics International 15: 96–99

Stavrakas P A, Sanders G T 1983 Sling support during pregnancy after hemipelvectomy: case report. Archives of Physical Medicine and Rehabilitation 64: 331–333

Stillwell A, Menelaus M B 1983 Walking ability in mature patients with spina bifida. Journal of Pediatric Orthopedics 3: 184–190

Varghese G, Hinterbuchner C, Mondall P, Sakuma J 1978 Rehabilitation outcome of patients with dual disability of hemiplegia and amputation. Archives of Physical Medicine and Rehabilitation 59: 121–123

Wood M R, Hunter G A, Millstein S G 1987 The value of stump split skin grafting following amputation for trauma in adult upper and lower limb amputees. Prosthetics and Orthotics International 11: 71–74

Appendix
General information and some helpful addresses

During the in-patient stage of rehabilitation the amputee generally receives help from the hospital social worker. This information and assistance usually consists of Social Service benefits, housing transfers, work availability, etc. Often, however, there are many obscure difficulties that arise after discharge, and generally it is the physiotherapist who is called upon to help, and in some cases supply information and addresses.

The following information and addresses may be of some use:

1. **NALD   National Association for Limbless Disabled**
   31 The Mall
   Ealing
   London W5 2PX

2. **BLESMA British Limbless Ex-Servicemen's Association**
   Frankland Moore House
   185 High Road
   Chadwell Heath
   Essex RM6 6NA

3. **REACH   The Association for Children with Hand or Arm Deficiency**
   13 Park Terrace
   Crimchard
   Chard
   Somerset TA20 1LA

4. **STEPS   The National Association for Families of Children with Congenital Abnormalities of the Lower Limb**
   15 Stratham Close
   Lymm
   Cheshire WA13 9NN

5. **The Thalidomide Trust**
   19 Upper Hall Park
   Berkhampstead
   Herts HP4 2NP

INFORMATION SERVICES FOR AMPUTEES

1. **Local Social Services Departments**
   These addresses can be located in local telephone books and will supply and give information covering: housing, aids and adaptations, education, benefits, employment, etc.

2. **RADAR The Royal Association for Disability and Rehabilitation**
   25 Mortimer Street
   London W1

3. **DLF   The Disabled Living Foundation**
   380–384 Harrow Road
   London W9 2HU
   One of many centres throughout the country.

4. **Citizens Advice Bureau**
   (address can be found in local telephone book)

INFORMATION SOURCES FOR PHYSIOTHERAPISTS

1. **ISPO International Society for Prosthetics and Orthotics**
   UK National Member Society Secretary
   Dr R. Platts
   Royal National Orthopaedic Hospital Trust
   Brockley Hill
   Stanmore
   Middlesex HA7 4LP

2. **National Centre for Training and Education in Prosthetics and Orthotics**
Curran Buildings
131 St James' Road
Glasgow G4 0LS
Scotland
RECAL — current awareness list is available for the above centre.

3. **The Chartered Society of Physiotherapy — Standards of Practice**, available from:
The Chartered Society of Physiotherapy
14 Bedford Row
London WC1R 4ED
A wide range of Standards, including Standards of Physiotherapy for the Management of Patients with Amputations.

4. **DSC Stores**
Physiotherapists should request lists of equipment available to amputees from local DSC stores, e.g. cramp-ons, antiperspirant spray for stumps, etc.

SUPPLIERS OF PROSTHETIC COMPONENTS

1. **C. A. Blatchford & Sons Ltd**
Lister Road
Basingstoke
Hants RG22 4AH

2. **Vessa Ltd**
Paper Mill Lane
Alton
Hants GU34 2PY

3. **Hosmer-Dorrance Corporation**
Address as for Vessa Ltd.

4. **Otto Bock Orthopaedic (UK) Ltd**
32 Parsonage Road
Englefield Green
Egham
Surrey TW20 0JW

5. **Hugh Steeper & Co. Ltd**
Roehampton DSC
London SW15 5PR

6. **LIC Care Ltd** (for the Femurett: see Ch. 5)
Princess Margaret Rose Orthopaedic Hospital
41–43 Frogston Road West
Edinburgh EH10 7AD
Scotland

7. **TWI-LITE**
Wellington House
1 Station Road
Heckington
Sleaford
Linconshire NG34 9JH

8. **Pillet Hand Prostheses Ltd**
Occupational Therapy Department
The London Hospital
Whitechapel
London E1 1BB

There are other prosthetic components available from many companies throughout the world which can be supplied in the UK, provided they comply with British Standards.

SPORTS ASSOCIATIONS

1. **BSAD British Sports Association for the Disabled**
34 Osnaburgh Street
London NW1 3ND

2. **BASA British Amputee Sports Association**
Ludwig Guttman Sports Centre
Harvey Road
Aylesbury
Berks HP22 7BR
Produce a newsletter with a great deal of information and are in contact with many other sports groups.

3. **The British Ski Club for the Disabled**
Stainforth Ski Centre
Hurst Road
Aldershot
Hants

4. **EAFA England Amputee Football Association**
Programme Director
Mr P. Stanyer
EAFA
64 Whitemoss Road

Blackley
Manchester M9 2LA

5. British Wheelchair Racing Association
20 High Point
Richmond Hill Road
Birmingham B15 3RU

6. The British Disabled Water Ski Association
18 Greville Park Avenue
Ashstead
Surrey KT2 2QS

7. Jubilee Sailing Trust Ltd
Test Road
Eastern Docks
Southampton SO1 1GG

8. Flying Scholarships for Disabled People
International Air Tattoo
Building 1108
Royal Air Force Fairford
Glos GL7 4DL

9. The British Federation of Disabled Cyclists
A. York
BCF
36 Rockingham Road
Kettering
Northants NN16 8HG

10. The National Handicapped Skiers Association
Mrs V. Peacock
Nash Dom
18 Barnett Park
Harlow
Essex CM19 4SD

11. National Handicapped Motorcyclists Association (Southeast)
81 Bracklesham Close
Farnborough
Hants GU14 8LP

12. The Society of One-Armed Golfers
D. Reid Honorary Secretary
11 Coldwell Lane
Felling
Tyne-and-Wear NE10 9EX

13. The National Association of Swimming Clubs for the Handicapped
Administrative Officer
Mrs Rosemary O'Leary
NASCH Administrative Office
The Old Tea House
The Square
Wickham
Hants PO17 5JT

TRAVEL ASSOCIATIONS AND INFORMATION

1. Disabled Drivers Association
Ashwell Thorpe
Norwich
NR6 1EX

2. Disabled Drivers Motor Club
Cottingham Way
Thrapston
Northants NN14 4LP

3. The BSM Disabled Drivers Training Centre
81–87 Hartfield Road
Wimbledon
London SW19

4. Banstead Mobility Centre
Damson Way
Orchard Hill
Queen Mary's Avenue
Carshalton
Surrey SM5 4NR

5. The Automobile Association — Guide for the Disabled 1992
(free for members, can be purchased)

6. Tripscope
63 Esmond Road
London W4 1SE
A telephone service providing free travel and transport information.

HOLIDAYS AND INFORMATION

Local Social Services departments and local councils generally have addresses and information.

1. **Holidays in the British Isles** and
Holidays Abroad can be obtained from the
publications department of RADAR:
Royal Association for Disability and Rehabilitation
25 Mortimer Street
London W1N 8AB

2. **Barrier-Free Scouting**
The Scout Association
Gilwell Park Training Centre
Chingford
London E4 7QW

3. **Disability Scotland**
Princes House
5 Shandwick Place
Edinburgh EH2 4RG
Has two holiday directors: one for Scotland
and one for the rest of the UK.

4. **Holiday Care Service**
2 Old Bank Chambers
Station Road
Horley
Surrey RH6 9HW

5. **The Winged Fellowship Trust**
Holidays for Disabled People
Angel House
Pentonville Road
London N1 9XD

MISCELLANEOUS ADDRESSES

1. **The Royal Horticultural Society**
80 Vincent Square
Horticultural Hall
London SW1P 2PB

2. **The National Trust**
36 Queen Anne's Gate
London SW1H 9AS

3. **The Society of Chiropodists**
53 Welbeck Street
London W1 7HE

4. **Horticultural Therapy**
Goulds Ground
Vallis Way
Frome
Somerset BA11 3DW

5. **PHAB Physically Handicapped and Able
Bodied Club**
12–14 London Road
Croydon
Surrey CR0 2TA

6. **SPOD Sexual and Personal Relationships
for Disabled People**
286 Camden Road
London N7 0BJ

Bibliography

Amputee rehabilitation

American Academy of Orthopaedic Surgeons 1965 Joint motion: method of measuring and recording. Churchill Livingstone, Edinburgh

Atkins D J, Meier R H 1988 Comprehensive management of the upper limb amputee. Springer-Verlag, New York

Banerjee S N 1982 Rehabilitation management of amputees, Williams and Wilkins, Baltimore

Coates H, King A 1982 Patient assessment: handbook for therapists. Churchill Livingstone, London

Croucher N 1981 Outdoor pursuits for disabled people. Woodhead Faulkner, Cambridge

Galley P M, Forster A L 1982 Human movement: an introductory text for physiotherapy students. Churchill Livingstone, Edinburgh

Ham R, Cotton L 1991 Limb amputation from aetiology to rehabilitation. Chapman and Hall, London

Humm W 1977 Rehabilitation of the lower limb amputee, 3rd edn. Baillière Tindall, London

Kostuik J P 1981 Amputation surgery and rehabilitation: the Toronto experience. Churchill Livingstone, Edinburgh

Kottke F J, Stillwell G K, Lehmann J F 1982 Krusen's handbook of physical medicine and rehabilitation, 3rd edn. W B Saunders, Philadelphia

Krueger D W (ed) 1984 Rehabilitation psychology: a comprehensive textbook. Aspen Systems, Maryland

Lamb D, Law H 1988 Upper limb deficiencies in children. Prosthetic, orthotic and surgical management. Little Brown, Boston

Macdonald EM (ed) 1976 Occupational therapy in rehabilitation, 4th edn. Baillière Tindall, London

Melzack R, Wall P 1982 The challenge of pain. Richard Clay (The Chaucer Press), Bungay

Mensch G 1987 Physical therapy management of lower extremity amputation. Heinemann Medical, London

Nichols P J R 1980 Rehabilitation medicine: the management of physical disabilities. Butterworth, London

Pendleton D, Hasler J (eds) 1983 Doctor and patient communication. Academic Press, London

Robertson E 1978 Rehabilitation of arm amputees and limb deficient children. Baillière Tindall, London

Rusk H 1977 Rehabilitation medicine, 4th edn. C V Mosby, St Louis

Saunders G T 1986 Lower limb amputations: a guide to rehabilitation. F A Davis, Philadelphia

Setoguchi Y, Rosenfelder R 1982 The limb deficient child. C C Thomas, Springfield

Troup I M, Wood M A 1982 Total care of the lower limb amputee. Pitman, London

Willard H S, Spackman C S 1971 Occupational Therapy, 4th edn. J B Lippincott, Philadelphia

Biomechanics and gait

Basmajian J V 1978 Muscles alive, 4th edn. Williams and Wilkins, Baltimore

Carlsoo S 1972 How man moves. Heinemann, London

Hughes J 1976 Human locomotion. In: Murdoch G (ed) The advance in orthotics. Edward Arnold, London, p 57–73

Hughes J, Paul J P, Kenedi R M 1970 Control and movement of the lower limb. In: Simpson D C (ed) Modern trends in biomechanics 1. Butterworth, London, p 147–179

Le Veau B 1977 Williams and Lissner — Biomechanics of human motion, 2nd edn. W B Saunders, Philadelphia

MacConaill M A, Basmajian J V 1969 Muscles and movement: a basic for human kinesiology. Williams and Wilkins, Baltimore

Rose G K, Butler P, Stallard J 1982 Gait: principles, biomechanics, and assessment. Orlau Publishing, Oswestry

Whittle M W 1991 Gait analysis: an introduction. Butterworth-Heinemann, London

Prosthetics

American Academy of Orthopaedic Surgeons 1981 Atlas of limb prosthetics: surgical and prosthetic principles. C V Mosby, St Louis

Department of Health and Social Security 1986 Amputation statistics for England, Wales and N. Ireland for the year 1985. DHSS, Norcross, Blackpool

Klopsteg P E, Wilson P D 1954 Human limbs and their substitutes. McGraw-Hill, New York

Mastro B A 1980 Elected reading: a review of orthotics and prosthetics. American Orthotic and Prosthetic Association, Washington

Murdoch G 1970 Prosthetic and orthotic practice. Edward Arnold, London

Murdoch G, Donovan R G (eds) 1988 Amputation surgery and lower limb prosthetics. Blackwell Scientific, Edinburgh

Phillips G 1990 Best foot forward. Granta Editions, Cambridge

Redhead R G, Day H J B, Marks L J, Lachmann S L 1991 Prescribing lower limb prostheses. Disablement Services Authority (from NHS Supplies Authority, Sheffield)

Royal College of Surgeons of England 1967 Symposium on limb ablation and limb replacement. Annals of the Royal College of Surgeons of England 40(4)

Vitali M, Andrews B G, Robinson K P, Harris E H 1986 Amputations and prostheses. Baillière Tindall, London

Wilson A B 1976 Limb prosthetics, 5th edn. Robert E Krieger, New York

Vascular disease, amputation

Abramson D I, Miller D S 1981 Vascular problems in musculoskeletal disorders of the limbs. Springer-Verlag, New York

Bloom A, Ireland J 1980 A colour atlas of diabetes. Wolfe Medical Publications, London

Burgess E M, Romano R L, Zettl C P 1969 The management of lower extremity amputations: surgery, immediate postsurgical prosthetic fitting, patient care. Veterans Administration, Washington

Faris I 1982 The management of the diabetic foot. Churchill Livingstone, Edinburgh

Gerhardt J J, King P S, Zett J H 1982 Amputations: immediate and early prosthetic management. Hans Huber, Bern

Gillis Leon 1954 Amputations. Heinemann, London

Greenhalgh R M (ed) 1985 Diagnostic techniques and assessment procedures in vascular surgery. Grune and Stratton, London

Levy W S 1983 Skin problems of the amputee. Warren H Green, St Louis

Little J M 1975 Major amputations for vascular disease. Churchill Livingstone, Edinburgh

Malt R A 1978 Surgical techniques illustrated 3(3). Amputations of the lower extremity. Little Brown, Boston

Siegfried J, Zimmermann M 1981 Phantom and stump pain. Springer-Verlag, Berlin

Walker W F 1980 A colour atlas of peripheral vascular disease. Wolfe Medical Publications, London

Warren R, Record E E 1967 Lower extremity amputation for arterial insufficiency. Little Brown, Boston

Equipment for disabled people

Department of Health 1990 The wheelchair training resource pack. Department of Health, Disablement Services Authority (available in every Health District/Board and Social Service Borough)

Equipment and services for people with disabilities. Health Publications Unit, Department of Health and the Central Office of Information

Male J, Massie B 1990 Choosing a wheelchair. The Royal Association for Disability and Rehabilitation (RADAR), London

Mandelstam M 1990 How to get equipment for disability. Jessica Kingsley Publishers and Kogan Page for the Disabled Living Foundation, London

Mary Marlborough Lodge 1988 Equipment for the disabled. Wheelchairs. Oxford Health Authority, Oxford

Tuttiet S 1990 Wheelchair cushions summary report, 2nd edn. Department of Health Disability Equipment Assessment Programme

Other

Coates T T 1983 Practical orthotics for chiropodists. Actinic Press, London

Coombs R, Friedlander G 1987 Bone tumour management. Butterworth, London

Croucher N 1989 Tales of many mountains. Amanda Press, London

Disabled Drivers' Motor Club Handbook 1985 Ins and outs of car choice: a guide for elderly and disabled people. Department of Transport, London

Goodwill C J, Chamberlain M A (eds) 1988 Rehabilitation of the physically disabled adult. Croom Helm, London

Hart E 1986 Victoria, my daughter: a true story of courage. Bodley Head, London

Jopling W H 1985 Handbook of leprosy, 3rd edn. Heinemann Medical, London

Klenerman L (ed) 1982 The foot and its disorders. Blackwell Scientific, London

Kohner N 1988 Caring at home. National Extension College, Cambridge

Maczka K 1990 Assessing physically disabled people at home. Chapman and Hall, London

Parkes C M 1972 Bereavement: studies in grief in adult life. Penguin, London

The Children's Act 1989 An introductory guide for the NHS. HMSO, London

Watson J M 1986 Essential action to minimise disability in leprosy patients. The Leprosy Mission, London

Watson J M 1986 Preventing disability in leprosy patients. The Leprosy Mission International, London

Wells P, Frampton V, Bowsher D 1987 Pain, management and control in physiotherapy. Heinemann Medical, London

Journals

Prosthetics and Orthotics International

Journal of Rehabilitation, Research and Development, Department of Veterans Affairs, Veterans Health Administration, Washington

For up-to-date information the Rehabilitation Engineering Current Awareness List can be obtained from:

The National Centre for Training & Education in Prosthetics & Orthotics
University of Strathclyde Curran Building
131 St James's Road
Glasgow G4 OLS

Index